SUSPENDED BODYWEIGHT TRAINING

SUSPENDED BODYWEIGHT TRAINING

Workout Programs for Total-Body Fitness

Kenneth Leung
with Lily Chou

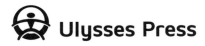 Ulysses Press

Published in the United States by
Ulysses Press
P.O. Box 3440
Berkeley, CA 94703
www.ulyssespress.com

ISBN: 978-1-61243-410-0
Library of Congress Control Number 2014943040

Printed in the United States by Bang Printing

10 9 8 7 6 5 4 3 2

Acquisitions: Keith Riegert
Managing editor: Claire Chun
Project editor: Lindsay Tamura
Editor: Lauren Harrison
Proofreader: Renee Rutledge
Indexer: Sayre Van Young
Front cover/interior design and layout: what!design @ whatweb.com
Cover photographs: studio © AYakovlev/shutterstock.com; woman © Rapt Productions
Interior photographs: © Rapt Productions except page 7 © Oleksandr Briagin/shutterstock.com, page 33 © holbox/shutterstock.com, page 59 © holbox/shutterstock.com
Models: Bryan Ausinheiler, Evan Clontz, Kenneth Leung

Distributed by Publishers Group West

Table of Contents

Part 1
OVERVIEW

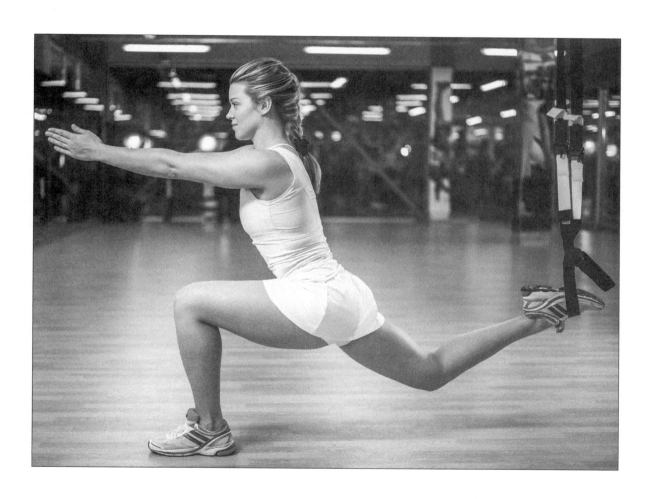

SUSPENDED BODYWEIGHT TRAINING: TAKING YOUR PERFORMANCE TO THE NEXT LEVEL

Every few years there seems to be a new fitness gadget in the gym that catches people's eyes. One of the more interesting ones to have come along is the suspended bodyweight trainer. Brands like TRX and Lifeline have reignited suspended bodyweight training, taking "old-school" exercises that were originally only done on rings by gymnasts and making them "new school."

There's a reason that almost every gym in America has added suspended bodyweight trainers. Suspended bodyweight training is both fun AND helpful. It turns stale exercises into challenging ones that will help rip your core. Even people who have no idea what they're doing can try one out and feel the burn in their abs and glutes. Just imagine what a little instruction and training can do!

If you're looking to learn more about suspended bodyweight training to enhance your exercise repertoire, you've come to the right place. This book will serve as a guide to using devices like the TRX, rings, and other suspended bodyweight straps and will provide examples and explanations of exercises that will help build strength, stability, and flexibility for personal benefit, as well as for a variety of sports.

Suspended bodyweight exercise is the cornerstone of many modern training programs for professional athletes in virtually every sport imaginable, including football, baseball, basketball, combat sports, triathlon, and swimming. Athletic programs worldwide use suspended bodyweight training to supplement their strength and conditioning routines, and with good reason—suspended bodyweight training is unique in that it challenges the stability of the performer, allowing you to improve your function through neuro-reeducation. By learning how to automatically stabilize your core, your apparent strength will surpass your previous plateaus. You'll become stronger and more toned, with a better overall build.

What's amazing about suspended bodyweight training is that anyone can do it. As a trainer for collegiate and professional athletes, I've used it to help give athletes more core feedback. As a physical therapist, I've used it to help make exercises easier for rehabilitating patients. Essentially, suspended bodyweight training allows you to instantly adjust an exercise's difficulty to whatever is most appropriate for your fitness level, whether you're a baby boomer who just wants to get up and down the stairs without pain or a college student who's working toward bulging biceps.

To give you a more meaningful workout, this book will help you understand basic exercise concepts. As an educator and a doctor of physical therapy, I try to make sure all of my patients know *why* they're doing something so that they can protect themselves from injury in the long run. By knowing and learning about suspended bodyweight training, you'll not only be able to ramp up the exercises as you progress, you'll also be able to modify them to fit your needs. With this book's easy-to-follow workouts and exercises with step-by-step instructions, you'll get not only what everyone wants, but what your trainer and physical therapist say you need: toned muscles, a strong core, flexibility, and, most importantly, a fun and challenging workout.

SO WHAT REALLY MAKES SUSPENDED BODYWEIGHT TRAINING DIFFERENT?

I'm one of the biggest cynics there is. Being in the fitness and health industry, I'm bombarded with the newest, craziest fads you can think of: supplements that will help you get ripped with minimal effort, diets that promise to make you as fit as a caveman, vibration plates that will shake your fat off, electrodes that will let you work out while you sleep, and even magic bracelets that claim to align your energy. Hey, if it works for you, that's great, but I don't want to waste my time with something that doesn't make sense and especially something that doesn't work better than the placebo effect.

What's the placebo effect? It's is when you believe something works—you'll have a psychological feeling that it's actually working, even if what you took (sugar pill, magic bean, etc.) was a total sham. I want something that really does work. I want something that has been *proven* with science to work. Not only that, I want something that I can feel working immediately. That's when I'll stick to it. With suspended bodyweight training, not only will you see results immediately or within the first few weeks, you'll continue to see gains in your training as you progress because of the amazing amount of flexibility and variability that you'll achieve.

When I first started using a suspended bodyweight trainer, it was just another toy. *Ok, cool, I can do this exercise and that one...not bad.* But the more I used it and the more familiar with it I became, I was able to do new exercises that worked my body like I had never felt before. My old workouts were like my first car: cheap but practical, and took me where I wanted to go. Adding suspended bodyweight training to my workout was like my dad giving me the keys to his brand-new BMW and saying, "Go crazy, son!" Now, all of a sudden, the good old push-up became a challenge again. I was able to add a ton of variety to my workouts, which not only made them a lot more fun, but worked my core at the same time. I guarantee that if you do the prone plank and jack knife exercise with a suspended bodyweight trainer, you'll feel your abs shredding and your fat burning in less time than it took you to read this paragraph.

Still skeptical? Find any certified exercise physiologist or your physical therapist and ask them about the importance of building a strong core and stability training. Read up on scientific journals that pick apart everything. While scientists can't agree 100 percent on global warming, all health practitioners agree that you need a strong core, which is key for decreasing lower-back pain and boosting sports performance.

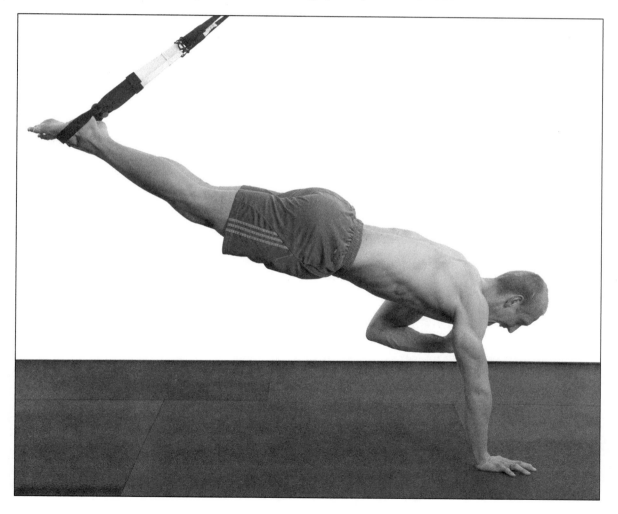

WHAT'S SUSPENDED BODYWEIGHT TRAINING?

Suspended bodyweight training is a way of using your bodyweight and gravity as the primary load for resistance. This means that you'll get all the resistance you'll need from your body alone. The beauty of suspended bodyweight training is that it can make your normal exercises both easier and harder. At its easiest settings, a suspended bodyweight trainer will make it easier to perform basic movements such as a squat. Can't do one push-up? No problem—use the suspended bodyweight trainer to take off 50 percent of your weight. Want to do 100 push-ups? Use the suspended bodyweight trainer to increase your load and instability, which will draw in more core muscles and strengthen your shoulder stabilizers. Now watch your performance improve.

Suspended bodyweight training is a type of instability training. By making you and your environment less stable, it requires you to self-stabilize, which draws in more muscles and increases their recruitment. The less inherently stable you are, the more you have to work to stay stable. Instability training has been shown to help prevent back, knee, and ankle injury. It works best as a supplement to your regular training by allowing you to have a low load on your spine while simultaneously forcing you to work your core muscles. Even the fittest athletes benefit from suspended bodyweight training as part of their warm-ups and during their off-season training.

Suspended bodyweight systems use non-elastic straps of varying length along with some kind of handle, whether it's just a rope tied into a circle or a fancy rubber handle. If you know what you want, you can make your own out of simple pieces of equipment. If you haven't used suspended bodyweight trainers regularly before, I'd recommend buying your own first or using them at the gym.

There are several brands of suspended bodyweight trainers on the market, including TRX, Power Systems Lifeline Jungle Gym, and GoFit Gravity Straps. When shopping for a suspended bodyweight training system, in addition to price, consider:

- **One anchor point vs. two:** Either is fine, but having one anchor point is slightly more convenient. The strap length is also easier to adjust and make both sides symmetrical, which will help to save a precious few seconds when trying to set up exercises in the middle of a workout.

- **Are the straps adjustable?:** Having straps that can change length is key to opening up the number of exercises that you can do and can also be used to change the difficulty level.

- **Handle type:** No loop, soft loop, or hard loop on the handle—having loops makes it easier for you to fit other body parts (e.g., your feet) into the suspended bodyweight device and can affect comfort. Soft loops are critical when packing the trainer into a small bag for travel, while hard loops may feel more comfortable on your extremities.

BENEFITS OF SUSPENDED BODYWEIGHT TRAINING

Suspended bodyweight training is versatile in that it allows you to adjust the difficulty level of many common exercises, optimizing the intensity and challenge for your specific needs. This way, you'll always have the perfect feedback. To truly understand how suspended bodyweight training can help you, it's best to understand the difference between strength and stability.

Most of us have an idea of what strength is. It's your ability to move an object, whether it be yourself or an external weight. The basic suspended bodyweight training exercises are great for building initial strength. What really makes suspended bodyweight training unique is its ability to help with a person's stability. Stability is similar to strength, but instead of your ability to move, it's your ability to resist movement. For example, when lifting an object from the floor, strength will allow you to resist gravity and pick up the object. Having stability will allow you to make it look easy and solid. It's stability that will keep your back in the optimal position so you can do the move over and over again without getting hurt. When you lack stability, you place a lot more stress and repetitive strain on your joints, which can lead to injury.

Most movements require both strength and stability. People get hurt and break down when an exercise demands too much of their body and they begin to lose stability. When your body and core are less stable, you'll suddenly find yourself with much less strength. The two go hand in hand and are complementary to each other.

Let's take the push-up as an example. The push-up requires you to first hold a plank position with your spine and keep your hips straight. Holding this position requires stability of your shoulders, trunk, and legs. As you drop down and do the push-up, you require shoulder strength to control the lowering and raising of your entire body. Throughout the whole motion, your body must stabilize and resist any bending or twisting that may occur. If your core isn't stable, your butt will stick up too far in the air and your back will sag, and everyone watching you will just shake their head. But when you work your core, you'll keep your body straight and aligned, and you'll make it look easy even if it isn't.

Now take another step up and add in suspended bodyweight training. If you put your feet into the straps, they're no longer locked to the ground—your legs might start swinging and so might your entire body. You have to suddenly divert your concentration and muscle energy toward resisting that swinging motion. The only things in contact with the ground are your hands, and so your wrists and your shoulders have to resist any side-to-side and rotational momentum from your body. You'll get a workout just trying to stay still! Now, take it up another notch and try the push-up. You'll have less overall muscle strength devoted to moving your body up and down because some of your muscles will be working extra hard just to stabilize everything.

After training with your feet in the straps, you'll find that doing regular push-ups on the ground is much easier than before—your body will have adapted and your natural stability will have improved. This will allow even more of your natural shoulder strength to be devoted simply to moving your body, which will result in exactly what we want: the ability to do more and better-looking push-ups.

In addition to strengthening your core and building stability, suspended bodyweight training is excellent for rehab and injury prevention. Working with unstable devices like BOSU balls, balance boards, and DynaDiscs is effective for reducing incidences of lower-back pain and improving stability in the knee and ankle joints. Suspended bodyweight training works in the same way by forcing you to self-stabilize your spine using your core musculature.

The following are more reasons why suspended bodyweight training is so great.

Versatility: Traditional exercises often require multiple dumbbell weights and other devices to provide variety. Purchasing your own set is great at first, but what happens after you get stronger and the weight you have is too light? One of the great benefits of suspended bodyweight training is that these exercises never become too easy. There's always a way to advance the exercise to make it harder without having to buy any extra equipment.

Unique stability training: With exercises, there are two types of movements: open-chain and closed-chain. Closed-chain exercises take place when your arms or feet are locked into the ground or something solid. Your limbs are inherently more stable, and you can generate more power. Open-chain movements occur when your limbs are free to move, such as your arm when throwing a baseball, or your leg in a taekwondo kick. Open-chain exercises require more inherent stability. This is why you can bench-press more total weight with a bar (closed-chain) than you can with individual dumbbells (open-chain). When trying to improve performance, it's best to do a combination of both types of exercises. With suspended bodyweight training, you can do both with just one piece of equipment.

Lightweight and compact: While almost every gym has caught on and provides a few suspended bodyweight trainers, hotel gyms are still lagging. However, since suspended bodyweight trainers are super-compact and light, you can pack them up and take them anywhere. Just connect them to any door or big tree and work out wherever and whenever you want.

Core engagement: Just about every suspended bodyweight exercise challenges your core more than its traditional counterpart. This means that you can do the same or similar exercise with a suspended bodyweight trainer for a shorter amount of time because you'll get a more dynamic and efficient workout more quickly.

It's fun: One underrated aspect of suspended bodyweight training is that it can be incredibly fun. Remember swinging on the swing set when you were a kid? There are exercises where you can use momentum and get the feel of swinging in the air. The unique challenge of suspended bodyweight training can't be replicated with traditional exercise equipment.

Anyone can use it: I've been going on about how I like to use suspended bodyweight training to boost my workouts and how challenging it can be for your core and crucial for power and stability. But suspended bodyweight training can be used on the other side of the spectrum, too. I regularly use it with my physical therapy patients to help make exercises easier as well. For instance, I use it to help people practice standing on one leg as well as make the squat easier to do. No matter what your age or level of fitness, you can use the suspended bodyweight trainer to boost your workout.

THE ANATOMY

In physical therapy, I like to tell people that almost everything begins with "the butt and the gut." It's not just a catchy phrase, though—it actually works. Almost every trainer and physical therapist knows that when helping an athlete improve their ankle flexibility or their recovery from an ACL injury, they *have* to train the glutes (the hip muscles) as well. Or if a pitcher is wearing out his elbow or shoulder, his rehab eventually takes him to his trunk flexibility. In anatomical terms, a simpler definition for a core muscle is any muscle that attaches to the spine.

When exercising, it's helpful to know which muscles are being emphasized. This allows you to fine-tune your exercise regimen to best meet your goals. The main muscles can be grouped into the following:

Trunk flexors: The abdominal muscles, including the rectus abdominis (the "six-pack muscle") and obliques.

Spinal extensors: The muscles, also known as the paraspinals, that run up and down your back.

Rotators and deep-trunk stabilizers: The multifidus, rotators, psoas, and transverse abdominis: These can be the most important—but also the most difficult—to train.

Pelvic: The butt contains the large muscles that are also the most fun to say—gluteus maximus and gluteus medius. But don't forget about the other hip rotators like the piriformis. In general, your hips are primary movers, which means they're responsible for generating the large forces necessary to move the entire body.

Shoulder: The trapezius (which has several parts), rhomboids, latissimus dorsi, and pectoralis major and minor. These muscles control the position of your scapula (shoulder blades) and contribute tremendously to your posture. Recruiting these muscles by packing your shoulders and arms can aid spinal stability.

By knowing which body part you want to emphasize, you can use the suspended bodyweight trainer in different ways. For instance, in the plank exercise, if you want to target the shoulders, you put your hands in the straps. If you want to target your abdominals or obliques instead, you put the straps around your feet and perform a prone crunch.

HOW SUSPENDED BODYWEIGHT TRAINING CHALLENGES THE CORE

When I first began learning martial arts, I was always told that my energy comes from within my belly. Even when I entered national competitions as a collegiate athlete, I didn't fully understand what this meant. But as I continued to train and attempted to get stronger and faster, I noticed that, by coordinating my trunk with my limbs, my movements became faster and stronger. By unleashing this potential, I was able to do quick and powerful movements such as speed breaks, which involve breaking a quarter-inch-thick piece of wood without anything supporting it (it's just dangling in the air).

Muscles and limbs don't work in isolation. With every arm movement, your trunk muscles are also activated. Rather than having your shoulders as the starting point of motion for your arms, you should have your trunk initiate it. You can see this with every functional movement. Let's look at a baseball pitch: The pitcher starts by facing sideways and lifts his front leg up. As he lunges forward, his pelvis turns and opens up, followed by his trunk, then shoulder, and, finally, the arm. In one quick, coordinated movement, the pitcher has used his entire body to throw a 5.5-ounce baseball.

Sitting in an exercise machine stabilizes your trunk and body. It's great for the exact opposite of what suspended bodyweight training is for: isolating your muscles. If you want to learn how to use everything together, you'll need to destabilize. By increasing the demand to your trunk stabilizers, you'll be able to recruit them even more during your functional movements, thereby increasing your apparent strength and performance simply with improved coordination and strength of your core without having to isolate each individual muscle.

Your core should always be active, whether you're performing the most basic of movements or the most complex. When you have a strong and functional core, your body serves as the stable platform from which your limbs move. When your body isn't stable or is weak, your arms and legs can't move as efficiently and you won't be able to reach your true potential.

Walking is pretty easy, right? We learn to walk before we can even remember anything. But it's actually a fairly complex motion of controlled falls that requires not only your legs but your entire trunk, head, and arms. When you walk, your hip muscles generate movement to help push your leg behind you. Simultaneously, your lower trunk muscles have to stabilize your spine to help carry your upper body forward. By keeping your trunk solid, you're preventing yourself from falling to one side. Muscles all the way up to your neck and shoulder blades also coordinate with each other to keep your head and arms in the right place.

In essence, your hips are the primary movers and are responsible for generating the large forces necessary to move your entire body. The lower trunk muscles, including your obliques and transverse abdominis (commonly known as TVA among trainers), and back musculature must be able to transfer all the movement generated by your hip muscles into the upper body. The trunk muscles do their best when they can work as stabilizers to prevent excessive movement of the spine, thereby preventing injury and wear and tear. The stronger and more stable your trunk is, the more force your arms and legs can generate.

To train your core muscles, it's important to remember that you don't have to actually make them move. Remember, stability is about your ability to *resist* movement. Take the plank exercise, for example: You're facedown and trying to prevent your hips and trunk from sagging. Your trunk muscles, especially those on the front of your body, are trying their best to keep your body from sagging and changing position. This is a great exercise for early and intermediate trunk strengthening.

But what about good old-fashioned sit-ups? Didn't everyone have to do them in their junior high fitness exam? The problem with the sit-up is that it encourages people to round their spine when, on average, people *don't* need more spinal flexion. People have flexed, rounded spines already from all the sitting that we do and from poor posture. Sit-ups and exercises that get us to round our back in a seated position also put a lot of stress on our discs, which can lead to more wear and tear on the spine and higher incidences of disc bulge and herniation.

The ideal exercises for beginners, rehabbers, and the average athlete are those that challenge the stability of our trunk. This is where suspended bodyweight training really shines. By making everything else unstable around you, your trunk muscles, especially the deep stabilizers, have to work much harder. Let's take a plank progression as an example:

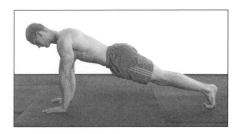

Plank with 2 hands and 2 feet on floor: Works both sides of your body evenly—you're stable and trying to prevent sagging.

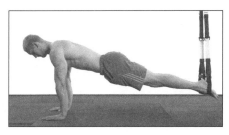

Plank with 2 hands on floor and 2 feet in suspended bodyweight trainer: Same as before, but now you may experience small movements because your feet might swing around. Your trunk and shoulders have to work harder to keep your feet stable.

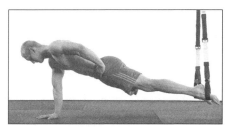

Plank with 1 hand on floor, 1 hand in air, and 2 feet in suspended bodyweight trainer: With only one hand on the floor, your trunk has to keep itself from falling down. You're also less stable.

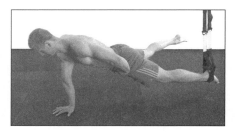

Plank with 1 hand on floor, 1 hand in air, 1 foot in suspended bodyweight trainer, and 1 foot in air: With only one leg on the floor, your body requires even more spinal stability than before. Everything is working, from your hip stabilizers to your trunk muscles and stabilizers to your shoulder stabilizers.

There are progressions and regressions for every exercise. Can't do a full plank but you want to challenge your rotational stability? Bend your knees and put your hands in the suspended bodyweight trainer. Or, if you're on the opposite end of the spectrum and you can now stabilize with minimal support (one arm, one leg), then do all that and move your hips or also do a one-handed push-up. In the end, the goal isn't to just be rock hard so that nothing can move your trunk. The real goal will be to move how you *want* to move and to be aware of what your trunk is doing. Maintain neutral spine (the natural curve of your spine) when you exercise; only move out of it when it's on purpose.

BEFORE YOU BEGIN

Suspended bodyweight training can be used by anyone and, with the proper steps, it's extremely safe. If you're recovering from an injury or surgery, consult with a medical professional prior to working out with a suspended bodyweight trainer. You can push yourself too hard and too early if you're still recovering from a surgery, so make sure you have given yourself enough time for your tissues to heal.

For everyone else, suspended bodyweight training is safe and appropriate as long as you take the normal, proper precautions before working out. If you have the strength to lean into a wall, you have the strength to perform suspended bodyweight training. If you're still not sure if suspended bodyweight training is appropriate for you, check with a local health professional who's familiar with suspended bodyweight training. Just because suspended bodyweight training can be used by anyone, that doesn't mean that every exercise can be done by every person.

Prior to purchasing a suspended bodyweight trainer, make sure you have a place in mind where you can attach it. Ideally, a solid anchor screwed into a ceiling or wall stud will give you the most options. Doors can be used as well once the area near the door is cleared. Always provide a sign on the other side of the door to prevent others from opening the door when you're exercising.

When you first grab onto a suspended bodyweight training device, you'll feel like a mess and wonder why your body won't stop shaking. However, just like with your regular exercises, you shouldn't experience any pain or symptoms from suspended bodyweight training. As you become stronger and more stable, you'll be able to use the device to make exercises even more challenging. Just be careful to know your limits—you won't benefit from exercises if they're *too* hard. Always make sure you have good form with your exercises before trying to make something more difficult.

SUSPENDED BODYWEIGHT TRAINING BASICS

Suspended bodyweight trainers can be set up indoors and outdoors once you have a grasp of what can serve as an anchor point (place where anchor is attached). Ideally, the anchor height or attachment point is anywhere from 6 to 9 feet high. You can still use suspended bodyweight trainers with heights that are lower or higher, but you'll have a different angle of pull. The setup may also create more swing than is desired.

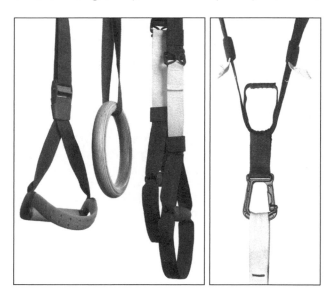

Outdoors, strong and sturdy overhanging tree branches are fun to work out with, but make sure they can support your full weight without bending. You can tie the suspended bodyweight trainer around the trunk as well and make it a "wall anchor." Indoors, ceiling mounts will allow more variation in exercise setup and are generally preferred when possible. Once you have a solid anchor point (or two, if you have two individual straps), test it by attaching your straps. At the lowest point, the straps should be around mid-calf length or 6 inches off the ground. Make sure that the setup can fully support your bodyweight before you begin your workout if you're hanging or pulling from it.

Most suspended bodyweight trainers come with setup instructions, but if you lose them or you made one on your own, always make sure that the attachment is secure. When attaching the suspended bodyweight trainer to the door, the preference would be to place the anchor on the side that the door opens so that it can't be pulled open by someone without them seeing the anchor.

When you're ready to use your suspended bodyweight trainer, once you hold the handles, pull back on the straps to remove any slack. The straps should be taut throughout the entire exercise.

KEY POSITIONS & POSTURAL CUES

When exercising, it's not so much what you do that's important, but *how* you do it. The best exercises in the world will only help you if you do them right. Likewise, doing them wrong can often lead to increased wear and tear on your body or, even worse, injury. One of the most important concepts to understand is how to protect your back.

Your back muscles and spine are at their strongest when they're in their middle position. This is called "neutral spine" and is a very common term among health professionals. In general, neutral spine represents the natural curve of your back and spine. When you stand tall, there should be a small concavity in the middle of your lower back. You can check by tilting your pelvis all the way forward and all the way back. Your back is in its strongest position when the curve is in the middle; that's when your joints and muscles are in the right place.

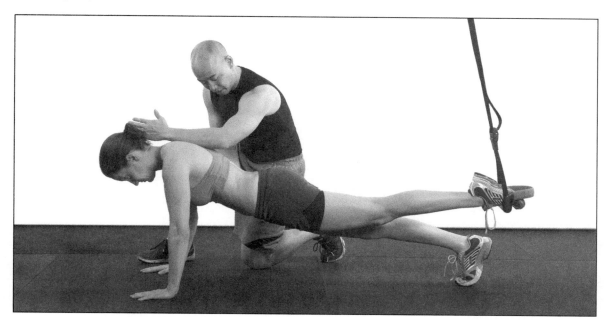

When you fully extend (bend backward) or fully flex (round or bend) your spine, your muscles are now at a disadvantage and cannot activate as well. Also, by being in an

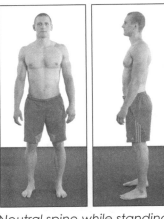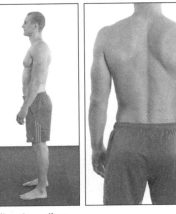

extreme position, you increase the stress to your back and risk of injury such as arthritis, nerve impingement, or disc herniation. So, in short, keep neutral spine for all of your basic strengthening exercises and you'll be safe.

Neutral spine while standing.

When you stand, the neutral spine position is usually obvious, but it becomes more difficult to maintain when you move your hips. When you do a proper hip hinge or deadlift, you should bend forward by driving your hips back while maintaining a neutral spine. If your back flattens, you might not feel pain, but that doesn't make it right! You also don't want to do the opposite and fully extend your spine because the increased concavity will lead to different kinds of pain (such as arthritis).

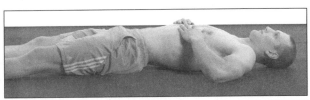

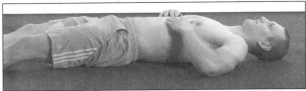

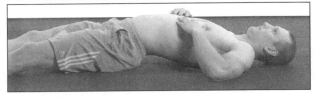

Top: Proper neutral spine while lying down. Middle: Flattened lower back (improper form). Bottom: Excessive arching (lordosis; improper form).

Another common mistake occurs when people do abdominal exercises on their back. If you were to keep neutral spine while on your back, your back should still have that same concavity and you should barely be able to slide your hand underneath the lower back. You should be able to maintain this same position when doing leg lifts, crunches, or any other diabolical ab exercise. It's even okay to place a small, rolled-up towel under the small of your back so you can push your back into it, but DON'T push your back into the floor. This is where you may hear disagreement among health professionals. By pushing your back into the floor, you're flattening out your spine.

If you're trying to strengthen your spine, why would you want to move it into a flattened, flexed position?

Moving your spine the opposite direction (arching it too much) is also improper. Commonly called "swayback," or excessive lordosis by physical therapists, this position can cause too much compression on the back parts of your spine, which can lead to excessive wear and tear on the joints of your spinal column.

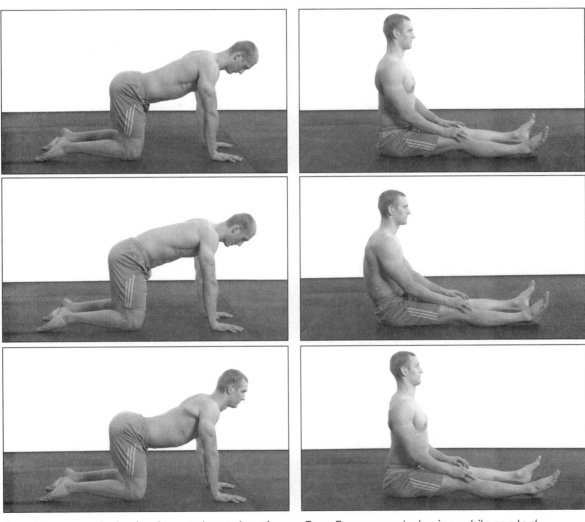

Top: Proper neutral spine in quadruped position (on hands and knees). Middle: Rounded lumbar spine (improper form). Bottom: Excessive arching (lordosis; improper form).

Top: Proper neutral spine while seated. Middle: Rounded back (improper form). Bottom: Excessive arching (lordosis; improper form).

Train your spine to be in neutral position during all of your motions. You'll feel the difference, and you'll protect your back. Take a look around at elite athletes, from a karate practitioner doing forms to a basketball player in a defensive stance to a powerlifter who's about to hoist a gargantuan weight—you'll notice that when they're about to exert themselves, they all have neutral spines. Of course, there are some exceptions to this rule. Some isolated sports-specific movements may require a non-neutral spine (the more common one being rowers in the catch position, or certain strong-man lifts that require you to wrap your body around a stone or get super low to flip a massive tire), but these involve an extra component of movement and flexibility.

BASIC EXERCISES

There are common exercise positions and movements that will be helpful with and without a suspended bodyweight trainer. Understanding how to do these exercises by themselves will speed up your comfort level with the suspended bodyweight trainer as well.

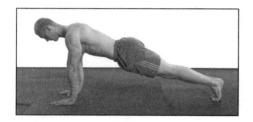

Plank: The plank is an exercise that will challenge the stability of your entire body. From your hands and knees (quadruped position), walk your hands out so that they're in line with your shoulders. Straighten your legs and maintain the same posture through your trunk as if you were standing tall. Keep your hips in line with your feet and shoulders. Remember to keep your neck and head in line with the rest of your spine. For increased emphasis on the core, squeeze your glutes to increase stability of your entire trunk. A common mistake is letting your butt sag.

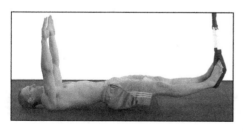

Supine Plank: Similar to the prone plank, the supine plank has you faceup with your heels or upper body resting on a slightly elevated surface (like a couch, bed, or suspended bodyweight trainer). You can fully lengthen your spine and hips so that only the back of your head and the backs of your shoulders are on the ground while your feet are elevated. Your back and butt should be working to stay straight and off the ground. Place your hands on the ground to assist with stability if necessary.

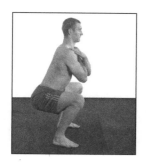

Squat: The squat is an excellent exercise when done correctly. Initiate the movement by simultaneously flexing your hips and knees. For the average squat, attempt to make your shins approximately parallel to your trunk. Make sure that as you flex your hips you don't round your spine, especially when you get as low as you can. Make sure you have no pain in your knees or anywhere else with this exercise.

OPTIMAL SQUAT FORM

One very common thing I hear from patients and some athletes is that they've been instructed to always keep their knees behind their toes during a squat. This kind of makes sense, right? The idea is to protect the knees. Well, I agree with one thing: You shouldn't have pain in your knees when you squat. And if there's pain in your knees, don't do anything that hurts them. If keeping your knees back helps, then do it. But if you have to keep your knees back when you squat, I wouldn't call it a true squat.

If you were to do a full squat to get your thighs parallel to the floor, just based off of simple biomechanics, any first-year biomechanical student can tell you that, for the average-proportioned individual, this is impossible to do while still keeping your knees behind your toes. In fact, you'll see a lot of people falling backward or having to pull their toes up to stop from doing so. This diverts energy and attention away from the squat movement. If you have to pull your toes up just to keep from falling backward, you're fighting against yourself.

To do a squat properly, your weight should be grounded through your feet right below your ankles. As your hips flex, your knees also flex. The knees should stay in line with the second toe on each foot while your feet remain flat on the ground. If there's no pain, go ahead and continue. Just make sure that your hips are moving back as well and engage *all* of your leg muscles to help you move that massive weight.

Hip Hinge: The focus of the hip hinge is to learn to move your hips without moving your trunk. When performed correctly, your leg and hip muscles, such as your gluteus maximus and your hamstrings, are the muscles that will power the hip hinge. Your back and trunk muscles will work to stabilize your trunk to prevent any extra motion. There are many great ways to learn the hip hinge, but often the simplest is the best: Focus on pushing your hips back while bending at the hips and keeping a neutral spine. You can use a dowel to align your spine.

When performed with a heavy load, the hip hinge exercise is commonly referred to as the "deadlift," for which there are also many variations. This resisted form of the hip hinge will help strengthen all of the muscles in your posterior, including your back, butt, and hamstrings.

BASIC STARTING POSITIONS WITH A SUSPENDED BODYWEIGHT TRAINER

Every exercise with the suspended bodyweight trainer will begin with one of the following eight positions. By familiarizing yourself with these positions, you'll be able to smoothly transition from exercise to exercise and can focus on each individual movement instead of setting up for it.

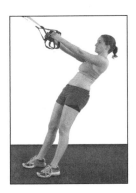

Standing Facing the Anchor: Grab the handles and step back until all the slack is removed from the suspended bodyweight trainer. Extend your arms and lean back. For increased intensity, step forward while maintaining tension on the straps.

Sample exercise: High Row (page 61)

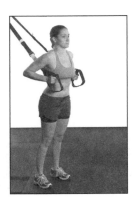

Standing Facing Away from the Anchor: Grab the handles and hold the straps in front of you. Step forward until slack is removed. If necessary, step back to increase the load onto the suspended bodyweight trainer.

Sample exercise: Pec Stretch (page 123)

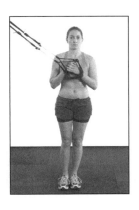

Standing Sideways from the Anchor: Grab the handles with one or two hands and face 90 degrees away from the anchor. Step away sideways from the anchor until the slack is removed and lean away from the anchor. Increase the difficulty by placing your feet closer to the anchor.

Sample exercise: Standing Hip Drop (page 99)

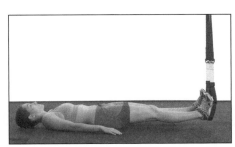

Lying Faceup, Feet in the Handles: Lengthen the straps and lie on the ground with your heels in the handles. To increase the pull from the suspended bodyweight trainer, move away from the anchor.

Sample exercise: Hamstring Curl (page 95)

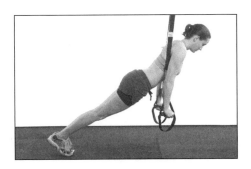

Lying Facedown, Hands in the Handles: Begin in the quadruped position with your knees and hands on the floor. With the straps lengthened, place your hands in the handles and then straighten out your legs and trunk to assume the prone plank position.

Sample exercise: Chest Press (page 65)

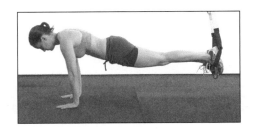

Lying Facedown, Feet in the Handles:

Option 1: Begin in the quadruped position with your feet toward the handles. With your knees on the ground, lift one leg and put it into the handle. Repeat with the other leg. Gently press your feet into the handles as you lift your knees off the ground and straighten your body. Attain the prone plank position with your feet in the straps.

Option 2: Sit facing the suspended bodyweight trainer. Place one foot through a strap. Lift your other leg over and place it through the other strap. Place weight onto the straps and follow the direction of the higher leg and turn over until you're facedown in the prone position.

Sample exercise: Push-Up with Feet in Straps (page 73)

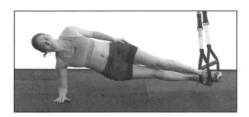

Lying on the Ground, on Your Side: This is similar to the prone position, but turn to the side instead of facing the ground. To emphasize your glutes more, place the bottom leg in the back.

Sample exercise: Side Plank (page 98)

PROGRESSING & REGRESSING EXERCISES ON THE FLY

There are several ways to increase or decrease the intensity of an exercise to make it the most appropriate for your skill set. Here are some basic rules for changing your intensity level.

Repetition: The easiest thing to do is simply to increase the number of repetitions (reps) that you do with each set of exercises. Depending on your goals, the optimal number of reps will vary. If you want more endurance, try a lighter resistance so that you can perform sets of 20. If you'd like to build more strength, aim to become fatigued with sets of 10 reps or fewer. *Note:* Exercising to the point of fatigue means that you perform repetitions of the same exercise until you can no longer complete them with ideal form. Performing half a rep or reps with suboptimal form not only teaches bad habits, but can be detrimental to your health!

Endurance/Time: An alternative to counting repetitions is to count by time. This is useful when performing exercises that require you to hold a position (such as the plank) and also useful when doing a circuit. Not having to count can help when you're quickly moving from one exercise to the next and you have enough thoughts running through your mind!

Rest Time: Optimal rest time can vary depending on your goals. When trying to boost your cardiovascular system, try shorter rest periods between sets, anywhere between 10 and 20 seconds. On the other end of the spectrum, when you're trying to build power (such as in your vertical jump), rest as much as you need to in order to recruit as much of your power as you can.

Speed: Changing the speed of movement doesn't necessarily make an exercise easier or harder, but it can help change your focus. When you need to improve your form and concentration, perform the exercise slowly so that you can correct your form while doing the movement. Once you're comfortable with the exercise, you can vary the speed of the movement to get the result that you want. For instance, I wouldn't train someone with depth box jumps until they could squat properly. Once an athlete can squat with good form at normal speed, I make it harder and have them do it with increased speed or momentum.

Base of Support: One subtle difference that you may not have noticed with regular exercises is your stance and base of support. Because suspended bodyweight training can make you less stable, it can exaggerate the amount of stability or instability that you use. Creating a wide base of support (hands or legs spread out on the floor) increases your stability—exercises will generally be easier in this position. Taking a narrow stance, or even using a single limb, makes your base of support much smaller and inherently less stable. This will require your trunk and body to stabilize more and will increase the difficulty of the movement. In addition, taking a staggered stance can make an exercise easier as this will allow you to change your pivot point.

Combine Movements: Once you're comfortable with an exercise, you can increase the variability by combining exercises. For instance, add spice to your push-up routine by trying to walk backward and forward on your hands after every few push-ups. With the power pull, hold a weight in your free hand and do a curl and press at the end of the movement. The combinations are endless!

Position: The position in which you set your body with respect to the anchor will make a dramatic difference in how hard you can make the exercise. Take the row, for example. It's often the first exercise that people try with a suspended bodyweight trainer, and making it easier and harder is just a matter of stepping backward or forward. When standing and facing the anchor, the farther back you set your feet, the more vertical you'll be;

you won't be able to lean as far back, and your legs will do most of the work of resisting gravity. To make it harder, simply inch your feet forward. If you walked your feet past the anchor point, you'd find that your arms will have to do all of the pulling (similar to an inverted row). With every exercise, the distance you set yourself from the anchor point will matter. If the resistance level isn't perfect right away, all you have to do is walk forward or backward until it is.

Part 2
WORKOUTS

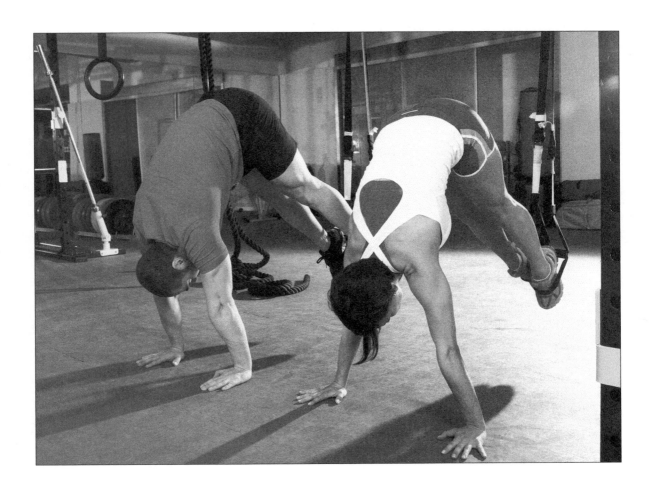

HOW TO USE THIS BOOK

In this section you'll find pre-set workouts to get you started, whether you're new to suspended bodyweight training or have been doing it for years. Some target areas of the body, while others are sport-specific to supplement your existing training regimen. These workouts aren't written in stone. They're meant to be basic building blocks for you to work from. You can swap in other exercises that you feel fit your needs more at any step. Once you're ready to design your own workout, see "Progressing & Regressing Exercises on the Fly" on page 30 for guidelines on customizing your program.

SAFETY

Make sure the anchor points are secure and that the straps can lock in place—there should be no "give" when pulling on the straps. With suspended bodyweight training, you're challenging your stability and balance, so make sure you're in an area where you can lie on the ground. When working out with others, make sure there's enough space between you and them so that you can all perform your exercises without interference from each other.

DESIGNING YOUR OWN WORKOUT

Once you're comfortable with some of the pre-set workouts and have an idea what exercises you like or need more of, you can devise your own personalized workout. When designing your workout, keep in mind what your goals are. Are you trying to build overall strength? Are you exercising to lose weight? Are you trying to improve your cardiovascular endurance? There are many different goals and thus just as many different ways to exercise.

For instance, a sprinter and a person trying to strengthen their legs to prevent lower-back pain can do the same lunge exercise but both have very different parameters. The person trying to build stability and strength to prevent lower-back pain should perform the lunge in a slow and controlled fashion, doing 3 sets of 10 reps, with each repetition optimized for form. A sprinter, on the other hand, has to focus on doing the same movement with maximum force output—she may choose to lunge down and up quickly and even add a jump. If her average race is 20 seconds, she can perform sets of 20 seconds to mimic her race demand.

When creating workouts for general fitness and conditioning, in the long run it's best to use a variety of tools and movements so that you can learn to adjust to any exercise. While you can create an entire workout with only suspended bodyweight trainers, ideally it's best to think of suspended bodyweight training as another tool in your expanded arsenal. From a total-body and total-function standpoint, suspended bodyweight training should be used in addition to free weights (heavy bars, kettlebells, dumbbells), plyometrics, and sport-specific exercises.

When focusing on an isolated movement or muscle group, try to make at least one of them incorporate a suspended bodyweight system. For instance, if my goal is to increase my pushing ability, I can rotate between sets of push-ups with my feet in the suspended bodyweight trainer, hands in the suspended bodyweight trainer, and then supine dumbbell presses. This will give me two kinds of closed-chain exercises with different types of stability demands, as well as an open-chain exercise (research shows that we benefit most from a combination of closed- and open-chain exercises).

That said, one of the biggest benefits of suspended bodyweight training is that you can do just about everything with it. So, when pressed for time or for ease and convenience, suspended bodyweight training is excellent because you can easily switch between different body parts or movements without having to walk across the room to grab another piece of equipment.

To help organize your exercise library, one method is to group exercises by function (hip hinging, squatting, pressing, pulling, and pushing). Another (simpler) method is to group by body part, which is how we categorize and group the exercises in this book. When organizing by body part, keep in mind that exercises may work multiple parts (one of the benefits of suspended bodyweight training).

The most important concept is to be mindful of your form or, more specifically, your ability to maintain your form as you fatigue. Suspended bodyweight training can make exercises easier and harder, so don't let the equipment distract you from what's really important: doing the exercises correctly. The best exercises are only helpful if you do them right. Feel free to exercise until exhaustion—just do all the movements with good form.

CUSTOMIZING THE EXERCISES TO YOUR FITNESS LEVEL

All exercises have numerous variations and I've included some of the more common ones. After becoming comfortable with the basic exercises, you can spice up your workouts by trying the suggested variations or making up your own. For instance, many standing exercises are described with your feet together. However, you can just as easily do these with your feet in a *staggered stance* (to make things easier) or with just *one leg on the ground* (to make things harder). See "Progressing & Regressing Exercises on the Fly" on page 30 for more examples on how to make an exercise or workout harder or easier.

GENERAL WORKOUTS

In the long run, having variability in your workouts is the best way to stay balanced. However, if you have specific goals in mind, such as strengthening your core or building explosiveness in your legs, then try these general workouts. Tiered levels of exercises are included for a wide range of abilities. If you've never done suspended bodyweight training, start with the beginner workouts (the first column of each workout). Once you get stronger and have adjusted to the difficulty level, you can progress to the intermediate and then the advanced workouts. If you're fit and have experience with instability and suspended bodyweight training, then you can try the advanced workouts.

Keep in mind that you may be advanced for some body parts and not for others so if you find that one exercise in a workout is a lot easier or harder than the others, there's nothing wrong with picking a variation that's more appropriate for your level. However, don't jump to the advanced workouts until you've mastered the basics and can maintain good form!

One last thing: The number of repetitions and sets are simply suggestions. Similar to the difficulty of the exercise, you can modify these to give you the proper intensity once you feel comfortable with the exercises.

LEGS

These exercises can be performed in a circuit, too—just do them back-to-back without rest. If you want to do more than one set, allow yourself a brief rest period after the last exercise if necessary.

BASE EXERCISE	BEGINNER	INTERMEDIATE	ADVANCED
Squat	Assisted Squat, *page 75* 10 reps	Y Squat, *page 60* 10 reps	Y Squat, *page 60* 10 reps
Hip Hinge	Hip Hinge, *page 91* 10 reps	Hip Hinge (Y variation), *page 91* 10 reps	Hip Hinge (Y variation), *page 91* 10 reps
Side Lunge	Assisted Side Lunge, *page 80* 10 reps each side	Assisted Side Lunge, *page 80* 10 reps each side	Abducted Lunge, *page 81* 10 reps each side
Pistol Squat	Assisted Pistol Squat, *page 89* 10 reps each side	Assisted Pistol Squat, *page 89* 10 reps each side	Pistol Squat (single-arm variation), *page 90* 10 reps each side
Knee Drive	Standing Knee Drive, *page 88* 10 reps each side	Front Single-Leg Hop, *page 84* 10 reps each side	Front Single-Leg Hop (air variation), *page 84* 10 reps each side
Lunge	Assisted Lunge, *page 76* 10 reps each side	Crossover Lunge, *page 100* 10 reps each side	Lunge with Lateral Reach, *page 78* 10 reps each side
Calves	Double-Heel Raise, *page 83* 10 reps	Heel Raise, *page 82* 10 reps each side	Single-Leg Calf Hop, *page 83* 10 reps each side
Bridge	Bridge, *page 93* 10 reps	Bridge (hands-free variation), *page 93* 10 reps	Bridge (single-leg variation), *page 93* 10 reps each side
Hamstring Curl	Hamstring Curl, *page 95* 10 reps	Hamstring Curl & Bridge, *page 96* 10 reps	Hamstring Curl (alternating variation), *page 95* 10 reps each side

ARMS & SHOULDERS

These exercises can be performed in a circuit, too—just do them back-to-back without rest. If you want to do more than one set, allow yourself a brief rest period after the last exercise if necessary.

BASE EXERCISE	BEGINNER	INTERMEDIATE	ADVANCED
Low Row	Low Row, *page 62* 10 reps	Low Row (walkout variation), *page 63* 10 reps	Deep Low Row (single-leg variation), *page 63* 10 reps each side
Biceps Curl	Biceps Curl, *page 69* 10 reps	Biceps Curl (single-arm variation), *page 69* 10 reps each side	Biceps Curl (single-arm variation), *page 69* 10 reps each side
Triceps Press	Triceps Press Elbow Extension, *page 71* 10 reps	Overhead Triceps Press Elbow Extension, *page 72* 10 reps	Overhead Triceps Press Elbow Extension (single-arm variation, *page 72* 10 reps each side
Chest Press	Chest Press (staggered stance), *page 65* 10 reps	Chest Press, *page 65* 10 reps	Chest Press (elbows-in variation), *page 65* 10 reps
L Deltoid Reverse Fly	L Deltoid Reverse Fly, *page 67* 10 reps	L Deltoid Reverse Fly (feet together), *page 67* 10 reps	L Deltoid Reverse Fly (foot position of choice), *page 67* 10 reps each side
Push-Up	Push-Up with Feet in Straps, *page 73* 10 reps	Push-Up (hands-in-straps variation), *page 73* 10 reps	Atomic Push-Up, *page 73* 10 reps
High Row	High Row, *page 61* 10 reps	Power Pull, *page 120* 10 reps each side	Power Pull with Overhead Press, *page 121* 10 reps each side
T & Y	T Fly (Reverse Fly), *page 68* 10 reps	X Reverse Fly, *page 64* 10 reps	Y Reverse Fly, *page 68* 10 reps

CORE

Attempt to maintain neutral spine as much as you can when performing each rep. Rest as much as you need to perform all exercises with good form. Aim to rest for 30 seconds or less.

BASE EXERCISE	BEGINNER	INTERMEDIATE	ADVANCED
Prone Crunch	Quadruped Hold, *page 101* 30 sec	Prone Crunch, *page 108* 30 sec	Prone Crunch, *page 108* 30 sec
Supine March	Supine March, *page 111* 30 sec	Supine March, *page 111* 30 sec	Supine March (double-leg variation), *page 111* 30 sec
Pike	Prone Crunch, *page 108* 30 sec	Pike, *page 109* 30 sec	Pike (shoulder-tap variation), *page 109* 30 sec
Hip Abduction	Standing Hip Drop (modification), *page 99* 30 sec	Standing Hip Drop, *page 99* 30 sec	Standing Hip Drop, *page 99* 30 sec
Quadruped	Quadruped with Leg Extension (forearm variation), *page 102* 30 sec	Quadruped with Leg Extension, *page 102* 30 sec	Suspended Quadruped with Leg Extension, *page 103* 30 sec each side
Side Plank	Side Plank (modification), *page 98* 3 x 10 sec each side	Side Plank, *page 98* 3 x 10 sec each side	Side Plank (thread-the-needle variation), *page 98* 3 x 10 sec each side
Mountain Climber	Mountain Climber, *page 110* 30 sec	Mountain Climber, *page 110* 30 sec	Mountain Climber (palm variation), *page 110* 20 sec each side
Supine Plank	Supine Plank, *page 94* 30 sec	Supine Hip Abduction, *page 97* 30 sec	Supine Hip Abduction (single-leg variation), *page 97* 30 sec
Plank	Plank (forearm variation), *page 105* 3 x 10 sec	Plank, *page 105* 30 sec	Plank Walk, *page 74* 30 sec

BALANCE

Balance involves our inner ear, eyes, and proprioception (our ability to feel where our limbs and joints are in space). Strength and coordination will help to maintain balance and help you recover when you trip. Our feet and hip strength are also very important. Perform each exercise with 10 seconds of rest in between, or just switch sides after each set.

BASE EXERCISE	BEGINNER	INTERMEDIATE	ADVANCED
Single-Leg Balance	Single-Leg Balance, *page 86* 30 sec each side	Single-Leg Balance, *page 86* 30 sec each side	Single-Leg Balance (eyes closed variation), *page 86* 30 sec each side
Standing March	Standing March, *page 87* 30 sec	Standing March, *page 87* 30 sec	Standing March (Y variation), *page 87* 30 sec
Heel Raise	Double-Heel Raise, *page 83* 30 sec	Heel Raise, *page 82* 30 sec	Heel Raise, *page 82* 30 sec
Hip Hinge	Basic Hip Hinge, *page 91* 30 sec	Single-Leg Hip Hinge, *page 92* 30 sec each side	Hip Hinge (Y variation), *page 91* 30 sec each side
Plank	Plank (forearm variation), *page 105* 30 sec	Plank, *page 105* 30 sec	Double-Limb Suspension Plank, *page 106* 30 sec
Side Lunge	Assisted Side Lunge, *page 80* 30 sec each side	Deep Assisted Side Lunge, *page 80* 30 sec each side	Abducted Lunge, *page 81* 30 sec each side
Supine Plank	Supine Plank, *page 94* 30 sec	Supine Plank (hands-free variation), *page 94* 30 sec	Supine Plank (hands-free variation), *page 94* 30 sec
Single-Leg Hip Hinge	Basic Hip Hinge, *page 91* 10 sec	Single-Leg Hip Hinge, *page 92* 20 sec	Single-Leg Hip Hinge, *page 92* 30 sec

LOWER BACK—FLEXIBILITY

For full mobility, it's important to stretch the joints above and below the lower back. Prior to beginning your stretches, it's essential to warm up properly. Hold all stretches for 30 seconds. For optimal gains, repeat each stretch 3 times.

BASE EXERCISE
Hamstring Stretch, *page 131*
Hip Flexor Stretch, *page 129*
Piriformis Stretch, *page 125*
Pec Stretch, *page 123*
Posterior Shoulder Stretch, *page 134*
Single-Arm Trunk Rotation, *page 128*

LOWER BACK — STRENGTH

A strong lower back is one that's stable and connects the forces generated from your legs up through your trunk to your hands. The expression "lift with your legs, not your back" is key here. You can only "lift with your legs" if your back is stable!

BASE EXERCISE	BEGINNER	INTERMEDIATE	ADVANCED
Squat	Assisted Squat, *page 75* 10 reps	Y Squat, *page 60* 10 reps	Y Squat, *page 60* 10 reps
Hip Hinge	Hip Hinge, *page 91* 10 reps	Hip Hinge (Y variation), *page 91* 10 reps	Hip Hinge (Y variation), *page 91* 10 reps
Resisted Rotation	Push Pull, *page 115* 10 reps	Resisted Trunk Rotation, *page 118* 10 reps	Resisted Trunk Rotation, *page 118* 10 reps
Quadruped	Quadruped with Leg Extension, *page 102* 10 reps each side	Quadruped with Leg Extension, *page 102* 10 reps each side	Suspended Quadruped with Leg Extension, *page 103* 10 reps each side
Plank	Plank (forearm variation), *page 105* 30 sec	Plank, *page 105* 30 sec	Double-Limb Suspension Plank, *page 106* 30 sec
Side Plank	Side Plank (top-leg-abducted variation), *page 98* 20 sec each side	Side Plank, *page 98* 20 sec each side	Side Plank (thread-the-needle variation), *page 98* 20 sec each side
Bridge	Bridge, *page 93* 10 reps	Bridge (hands-free variation), *page 93* 10 reps	Bridge (marching variation), *page 93* 10 reps
Supine Plank	Supine Plank, *page 94* 30 sec	Supine Plank (hands-free variation), *page 94* 30 sec	Supine Hip Abduction, *page 97* 30 sec
Hamstring Curl	Hamstring Curl, *page 95* 10 reps	Hamstring Curl (hands-free variation), *page 95* 10 reps	Hamstring Curl & Bridge, *page 96* 10 reps

TOTAL-BODY CONDITIONING

Do exercises 1, 2, and 3 and then repeat for 3 sets. Then move on to 4, 5, and 6 and repeat for 3 sets. Finish with 7, 8, and 9 for 3 sets. Begin with 30 seconds per exercise with 15 seconds of rest. Progress by either increasing each set time or decreasing your rest time.

BASE EXERCISE	BEGINNER	INTERMEDIATE	ADVANCED
Hip Hinge	Hip Hinge, *page 91* 10 reps	Hip Hinge (Y variation), *page 91* 10 reps	Hip Hinge (Y variation), *page 91* 10 reps
Power Pull	Low Row (single-arm variation), *page 63* 5 reps each side	Power Pull (staggered stance), *page 120* 5 reps each side	Power Pull, *page 120* 5 reps each side
Triceps Press Elbow Extension	Triceps Press Elbow Extension (high position), *page 71* 10 reps	Triceps Press Elbow Extension (middle position), *page 71* 10 reps	Triceps Press Elbow Extension (low position), *page 71* 10 reps
Squat	Assisted Squat, *page 75* 10 reps	Assisted Squat (forward lean variation), *page 75* 10 reps	Y Squat, *page 60* 10 reps
Row + Biceps Curl	Row + Biceps Curl (staggered stance), *page 69* 10 reps	Row + Biceps Curl, *page 69* 10 reps	Row + Biceps Curl (single-leg stance), *page 69* 10 reps
Mountain Climber	Mountain Climber, *page 110* 30 sec	Mountain Climber (2 feet away), *page 110* 30 sec	Mountain Climber (4 feet away), *page 110* 30 sec
Lunge	Assisted Lunge, *page 76* 10 reps	Assisted Side Lunge, *page 80* 10 reps	Lunge with Lateral Reach, *page 78* 10 reps
Trunk Rotation	Resisted Trunk Rotation, *page 118* 10 reps	Resisted Trunk Rotation, *page 118* 10 reps	Resisted Trunk Rotation, *page 118* 10 reps
Crunch & Push-Up	Plank, *page 105* 30 sec	Prone Crunch, *page 108* 30 sec	Atomic Push-Up, *page 73* 30 sec

CARDIO

Some of these exercises are intense, so make sure you give yourself enough rest before moving on to the next. Always maintain a stable trunk and a neutral spine when performing each exercise.

BASE EXERCISE	BEGINNER	INTERMEDIATE	ADVANCED
March	Standing March, *page 87* 30 sec	Standing Knee Drive (cardio jog variation), *page 88* 30 sec	Standing Knee Drive (cardio sprint variation), *page 88* 30 sec
Front Single-Leg Hop	Front Single-Leg Hop, *page 84* 30 sec each side	Front Single-Leg Hop, *page 84* 30 sec each side	Front Single-Leg Hop (air variation), *page 84* 30 sec each side
Row	Low Row, *page 62* 10 reps	High Row, *page 61* 10 reps	X Reverse Fly, *page 64* 10 reps
Crossover Lunge	Crossover Lunge, *page 100* 30 sec	Crossover Lunge (skater variation), *page 100* 30 sec	Crossover Lunge (skater variation), *page 100* 30 sec
Squat	Assisted Squat, *page 75* 10 reps	Assisted Squat (forward lean variation), *page 75* 10 reps	Assisted Squat (jump variation), *page 75* 10 reps
Mountain Climber	Mountain Climber, *page 110* 10 reps each side	Mountain Climber, *page 110* 15 reps each side	Mountain Climber, *page 110* 20 reps each side
Lunge	Lunge, *page 77* 10 reps each side	Lunge (jump variation), *page 77* 10 reps each side	Lunge (jump variation), *page 77* 10 reps each side
Plank	Plank, *page 105* 30 sec	Prone Crunch, *page 108* 30 sec	Atomic Push-Up, *page 73* 30 sec

SPORT-SPECIFIC WORKOUTS

Because there are so many movements and challenges that each individual sport requires, a unique combination of flexibility, strength, and control is needed for each one. Suspended bodyweight training is a great way to supplement your regular training routine. You'll find suggested suspended training workouts for a variety of sports in this section.

For many sports that involve ankle injuries, increasing foot strength and balance will help decrease the likelihood of ankle sprains. What isn't as commonly known is that it's also important to have good hip and trunk stability, which can help with balance. Frontal plane control is a common concept with many of these sports. Being strong in the frontal plane means having good control and strength with "abduction." This directly leads to lateral agility and control, especially when you're on one leg.

The reps and sets provided in the following workouts are purely estimates. When considering injury prevention, the most important factor is form. Make sure that every repetition is performed well. Practice doesn't make perfect—perfect practice makes perfect!

Before performing your training routine, warm up properly to increase your blood flow and flexibility. Perform any full-body explosive movements (such as sprints and heavy lifts that require perfect form, like snatches) first. Then focus on strengthening exercises, incorporating the suspended training exercises suggested in this book. If your range of motion is limited, you can perform stretches after warming up. Otherwise, save the heavy stretching for the end of your workout to decrease soreness.

Please note that, while suspended bodyweight training is an excellent overall tool, athletes looking for a truly elite and well-balanced exercise routine will need to perform a couple of exercises without any suspension, which is why squats and deadlifts (or hinges) are included in some of these workouts. Once you get the form down, it's time to add weight, be it a bar, dumbbells, kettlebells, or sandbags. Of course, with increased weight, there's decreased margin for error. Always consult with a trainer or physical therapist if you're not sure of your form.

Please refer to page 27 for proper squat form. Some other key tips: line up your knees and align them with your second toe; focus your weight on your heels, just in front of the ankle joint; actively push your butt back at the bottom of the squat to keep your spine neutral.

The hip hinge, or deadlift, is my favorite exercise for building up a strong butt, back, and hamstrings. It's also great for helping develop good posture. The key is to make sure that your spine is in neutral, meaning that you maintain the small slight curve of your lower back. You may use a stick to help practice doing the hip hinge. See the basic Hip Hinge on page 91 for instructions on how to do this version without weights.

BASEBALL

Many injuries in baseball are a direct result of the repetitive physical demands that the sport places on its athletes. To launch a baseball 90 mph or more, a pitcher must wind up and contort his body to transmit all of his body's speed and power into his throwing arm. By developing the proper flexibility to get into the cocked position and the necessary strength in the core and shoulder, many injuries can be prevented.

A baseball pitch typically starts with a windup that involves full trunk rotation and external rotation of the shoulder. As the pitcher uncoils his body, the ball is launched out of his hand after the entire body has already moved toward the plate. This can put stress along the different body parts that are transferring the energy, including the obliques, the shoulder, and the inside elbow. Finally, to stop the movement, the rotator cuff and posterior shoulder must stop the arm's momentum.

Common Preventable Injuries: Little League elbow, rotator cuff strain, quadriceps and hamstrings strain, oblique strain

Physical Demands: shoulder flexibility, quick starts and stops, trunk rotation

Goals of Program: grip strength, shoulder and trunk strength

EXERCISE	REPS/DURATION
Torso Twist, *page 127*	3 x 10 reps
Single-Leg Hip Hinge, *page 92*	3 x 10 reps
Side Plank, *page 98*	3 x 30 sec
Bridge (single-leg variation), *page 93*	3 x 10 reps
L Deltoid Reverse Fly, *page 67*	3 x 20 reps
Power Pull, *page 120*	3 x 10 reps
Prone Oblique Crunch, *page 112*	3 x 30 sec each side
Hamstring Curl, *page 95*	3 x 20 reps

BASKETBALL

In basketball, ankle sprains commonly occur from the frequent changes in direction, as well as from jumping and landing, whether on the floor or on another player's foot. While balance and footwork are necessary, building endurance and proper conditioning will help prevent further injury (more injuries happen in the second half of a game than the first).

Common Preventable Injuries: knee pain, ankle sprain, flagging endurance/fatigue

Physical Demands: jumping power, frontal plane control, trunk and shoulder flexibility, hip strength

Goals of Program: ankle flexibility, frontal plane control

EXERCISE	REPS/DURATION
Front Single-Leg Hop, *page 84*	3 x 60 sec
Single-Leg Hip Hinge, *page 92*	3 x 10 reps
Abducted Lunge, *page 81*	3 x 10 reps
Resisted Trunk Rotation, *page 118*	3 x 10 reps
Reverse Plank Walk, *page 74*	3 x 5 reps
Bridge, *page 93*	3 x 20 reps
Mountain Climber, *page 110*	3 x 30 sec

BOXING

What's the one exercise that you always see boxers do? Jump rope. Why? Because boxers need to stay mobile in order to dart in and out of punching range. The next in-demand ability isn't as obvious: trunk strength. Your trunk is what enables all the power from your legs to transfer into your fists. Except for the jab, every punch, from hooks to uppercuts, requires a boxer to use his entire body to land power behind those fists.

Physical Demands: cardio, footwork, shoulder strength

Goals of Program: shoulder strength, trunk strength

EXERCISE	REPS/DURATION
High Row, *page 61*	3 x 10 reps
Push-Up with Feet in Straps, *page 73*	3 x 20 reps
Front Single-Leg Hop (air variation), *page 84*	3 x 60 reps each side
Supine March (double-leg variation), *page 111*	3 x 60 sec
Mountain Climber, *page 110*	3 x 60 sec
Bridge (single-leg variation), *page 93*	3 x 20 reps
Prone Oblique Crunch, *page 112*	3 x 60 sec

FOOTBALL

Like other sports that demand frequent changes in direction, football results in players dealing with ankle and knee ligament sprains. For conditioning and leverage, it's important to have mobile hips to keep your center of mass low. Developing strong legs will allow a lineman to take advantage of a lower center of mass. Position players need to be able to cut sharply and change direction, while quarterbacks need a strong and flexible shoulder. Modify your training regimen based on the specific demands of the position you play. Traditional football conditioning involves powerlifts and other explosive movements. Supplement this with movements and exercises that challenge one limb at a time when upright. This will improve your ability to move in the frontal plane and improve your lateral agility and control.

Note: Prior to performing any explosive workout, always remember to properly warm up. Perform agility work that mimics the footwork demanded by your position (cone and shuttle drills), followed by a quick sprint workout. Then perform power lifts. Supplement the workout with these suspension-assisted exercises to help with leg flexibility and strength.

Common Preventable Injuries: hamstring strain, ankle sprain, knee ligament sprain

Physical Demands: explosive leg strength, frontal plane strength

Goals of Program: ankle flexibility, frontal plane control

EXERCISE	REPS/DURATION
Abducted Lunge, *page 81*	3 x 10 reps
Pistol Squat, *page 90*	3 x 10 reps each side
Hamstring Curl, *page 95*	3 x 20 reps
Crossover Lunge, *page 100*	3 x 10 reps
Mountain Climber, *page 110*	10 x 10 sec

GOLF

Often underestimated, golf can demand a lot of physical power and flexibility. Rotational power for golf swings comes from a solid trunk, strength in the hips, and flexibility in the shoulders. When you're lacking any one of these attributes, you'll have to compensate and "cheat," which can lead to injury. Two levels of workouts are suggested here. If you're new to golf and/or lack shoulder flexibility and hip strength, try the beginner workout first. The advanced workout is to help maintain the flexibility that a golfer needs, as well as add power for longer drives.

Common Preventable Injuries: lower-back sprains and strains, shoulder impingement, knee pain

Physical Demands: hip flexibility, trunk rotation, trunk strength

Goals of Program: trunk and hip flexibility, shoulder flexibility, hip strength

BEGINNER	ADVANCED
Torso Twist, *page 127* 10 reps	Torso Twist, *page 127* 10 reps
Hip Hinge, *page 91* 10 reps	Single-Leg Hip Hinge, *page 92* 10 reps
Pec Stretch, *page 123* 20 sec	Pec Stretch, *page 123* 20 sec
Posterior Shoulder Stretch, *page 134* 20 sec	Posterior Shoulder Stretch, *page 134* 20 sec
Bridge, *page 93* 10 reps	Bridge (single-leg variation), *page 93* 10 reps
Push Pull, *page 115* 10 reps each side	Concentric Trunk Rotation, *page 117* 10 reps each side
Assisted Side Lunge, *page 80* 10 reps each side	Crossover Lunge, *page 100* 10 reps each side
Piriformis Stretch, *page 125* 20 sec	Piriformis Stretch, *page 125* 20 sec

ROWING

The entire posterior chain is repeatedly stressed during the rowing motion. Rowers need to have extremely strong and durable backs, shoulders, and even forearms to meet the demands of the sport. When one part of the body is weak, adjacent body parts will compensate for the weakness, which may lead to injuries in those areas. In addition to strength, having proper flexibility of all the joints in the legs will help with maintaining ideal form.

The row is a unique movement in which it's acceptable to round your lower back. At the catch position (the moment the blade enters the water), the arms are straight and the back should be firm. This will allow the power to come from the legs. Having adequate hip flexion will assist with decreasing stress to the back. Make sure the knees are in line with the feet and hips (you don't want them pointing inward). The arms should slowly take over only after the leg drive is near complete.

Common Preventable Injuries: wrist extensor tendinitis, rib fracture, lower-back pain, knee pain

Physical Demands: grip strength, ankle flexibility, hip flexibility

Goals of Program: back and hip strength

EXERCISE	REPS/DURATION
Hip Hinge, *page 91*	3 x 10 reps
Assisted Squat, *page 75*	3 x 10 reps
Basic Hip Hinge, *page 91*	3 x 5 reps
Side Plank, *page 98*	3 x 60 sec
Bridge (single-leg variation), *page 93*	3 x 20 reps
High Row, *page 61*	3 x 20 reps
Power Pull, *page 120*	3 x 10 reps
Hip Flexor Stretch, *page 129*	3 x 30 sec
Calf Stretch (soleus/ankle variation), *page 130*	3 x 30 sec

RUNNING

While running is one of the most popular sports among amateurs, it can be challenging to the body. Many runners have similar injuries that can be minimized with a proper complementary strengthening program. Strong lateral stabilizers as well as calves and hamstrings are important when running. This workout requires more frequent repetitions because most recreational runners need endurance. Because of the high variability of conditioning levels, three levels of suggested exercises are provided.

Common Preventable Injuries: patello-femoral pain, foot and ankle tendinopathy, lower-back pain

Physical Demands: lateral hip strength, foot strength

Goals of Program: hip, knee, and ankle strength for proper running mechanics

BASE EXERCISE	BEGINNER	INTERMEDIATE	ADVANCED
Calves	Double-Heel Raise, *page 83* 3 x 10 reps	Heel Raise, *page 82* 3 x 10 reps each side	Single-Leg Calf Hop, *page 83* 3 x 10 reps each side
Front Single-Leg Hop	Front Single-Leg Hop, *page 84* 20 reps each side	Front Single-Leg Hop (air variation), *page 84* 20 reps each side	Front Single-Leg Hop (air variation), *page 84* 20 reps each side
Lunge	Assisted Lunge, *page 76* 10 reps each side	Crossover Lunge, *page 100* 10 reps each side	Lunge (jump variation), *page 77* 10 reps each side
Squat	Assisted Pistol Squat, *page 89* 10 reps each side	Assisted Pistol Squat (single-arm variation), *page 89* 10 reps each side	Assisted Pistol Squat (single-arm variation), *page 89* 10 reps each side
Standing Knee Drive	Standing Knee Drive, *page 88* 30 sec	Standing Knee Drive (cardio jog variation), *page 88* 30 sec	Standing Knee Drive (cardio sprint variation), *page 88* 30 sec
Mountain Climber	Prone Crunch, *page 108* 30 sec	Mountain Climber, *page 110* 30 sec	Mountain Climber (palm variation), *page 110* 30 sec
Hamstring Curl	Hamstring Curl, *page 95* 20 reps	Hamstring Curl (hands-free variation), *page 95* 20 reps	Hamstring Curl (alternating variation), *page 95* 20 reps each side
Bridge	Bridge, *page 93* 20 reps	Bridge (single-leg variation), *page 93* 20 reps	Bridge (single-leg variation), *page 93* 20 reps
Side Plank	Side Plank (modification), *page 98* 3 x 10 sec each side	Side Plank, *page 98* 5 x 10 sec each side	Side Plank (top-leg-abducted variation), *page 98* 5 x 10 sec each side

SOCCER

Ankle sprains and ACL tears are the most common injuries in soccer. Since these occur in the lower joints, having excellent lower-body proprioception and control will help prevent non-contact injuries. Make sure to strengthen the legs in every direction, especially sideways (in the frontal plane) to help with agility, cutting, and swift changes in direction.

Common Preventable Injuries: ankle sprain, hamstring pull, ACL tear, Achilles tendinitis, IT band syndrome

Physical Demands: foot and ankle strength, endurance, leg strength

Goals of Program: ankle flexibility, explosive leg strength, hip strength, ankle flexibility, lateral hip strength, frontal plane control, calf strength

EXERCISE	REPS/DURATION
Single-Leg Balance, *page 86*	3 x 30 sec
Basic Hip Hinge, *page 91*	3 x 10 reps
Abducted Lunge, *page 81*	3 x 10 reps
Side Plank, *page 98*	3 x 60 sec
Pistol Squat, *page 90*	3 x 10 reps
Mountain Climber, *page 110*	3 x 60 sec
Hamstring Curl, *page 95*	3 x 20 reps
Calf Stretch, *page 130*	3 x 30 sec

SWIMMING

With any sport that demands a repetitive motion, having proper form is key. In addition, a flexible trunk that allows you to fully rotate will help prevent both shoulder and neck strain and allow your shoulders to work more efficiently.

When performing the crawl, having increased trunk rotation helps significantly with two things: It allows your head to rotate farther to the side when breathing without having to extend your neck, and it allows you to clear your arm and shoulder out of the water. With increased trunk rotation, you'll have a more powerful stroke without fatiguing your arm muscles as much. Breaststroker's knee, when the medial (inside) part of the knee becomes inflamed, is a common injury. Make sure to give yourself adequate rest and to switch strokes. To increase the lateral stability of the knee, perform single-leg exercises that challenge frontal plane stability.

Common Preventable Injuries: shoulder strain, lower-back strain, neck strain, knee strain

Physical Demands: upper-trunk flexibility, hip flexibility

Goals of Program: trunk flexibility and strength, shoulder flexibility

EXERCISE	REPS/DURATION
Single-Arm Trunk Rotation, *page 128*	3 x 30 sec
Single-Leg Hip Hinge, *page 92*	3 x 10 reps
High Row, *page 61*	3 x 20 reps
Abducted Lunge, *page 81*	3 x 20 reps
Power Pull, *page 120*	3 x 10 reps
Plank Walk, *page 74*	3 x 5 reps
L Deltoid Reverse Fly, *page 67*	3 x 20 reps
Concentic Trunk Rotation, *page 117*	3 x 10 reps
X Reverse Fly, *page 64*	3 x fatigue
Hip Flexor Stretch, *page 129*	3 x 30 sec

TENNIS

In addition to requiring proper grip on the racquet and good form, tennis can be very demanding on the body. Many racquet sports require proper grip to reduce stress on the wrist and forearm; swings that come primarily from the wrist will put unnecessary stress on the forearm. Good trunk and shoulder flexibility goes a long way toward protecting the elbow and back. In addition, the constant shifts in direction require solid hip and leg strength.

The tennis serve requires you to wind up your body so that the rear shoulder and arm can swing forward. When the shoulder lacks the ability to be pulled back, you must compensate. This leads to increased strain on the back, shoulder, and elbow. To help with this, ensure that you have as much mobility in your upper trunk as possible. This will help you to pull your shoulder blade back, which will allow you to wind up for your serve.

Tip: Planks can be a great way to increase wrist flexibility and strength. However, only perform them on your palms if your wrists don't hurt. You can slowly increase your tolerance to them with each workout.

Common Preventable Injuries: elbow and forearm pain, rotator cuff and shoulder pain, knee pain, back pain, ankle sprain, calf strain

Physical Demands: trunk rotation, shoulder flexibility

Goals of Program: ankle flexibility, frontal plane control

EXERCISE	REPS/DURATION
Assisted Squat, *page 75*	3 x 10 reps
Hip Hinge (Y variation), *page 91*	3 x 5 reps
Assisted Side Lunge, *page 80*	3 x 10 reps
Power Pull, *page 120*	3 x 10 reps
Low Row (single-arm variation), *page 63*	3 x 10 reps
Single-Arm Trunk Rotation, *page 128*	3 x 10 reps
Side Plank (thread-the-needle variation), *page 98*	3 x 30 sec
L Deltoid Reverse Fly, *page 67*	3 x 20 reps
Plank, *page 105*	3 x 30 sec
Single-Arm Trunk Rotation, *page 128*	3 x 30 sec
Pec Stretch, *page 123*	3 x 30 sec

WRESTLING

The combination of leverage and twisting that occurs during matches places a lot of stress on the shoulder, making shoulder dislocation one of the more common injuries that wrestlers and grapplers experience. To help prevent this, it's important to develop strength in the shoulder *and* flexibility in the trunk and entire shoulder girdle. The unique motions of grappling also emphasize core strength through a wide range of motions. Perform abdominal strengthening from varying positions (for instance, instead of just planks, perform them with knee crunches to alternate shoulders).

Tip: Make sure not to hyperextend your elbows when supporting your weight through your arms. For improved neck strength, keep your chin tucked in with all exercises.

While most core exercises demand keeping your spine in neutral, you can modify these exercises to simulate common grappling maneuvers. For example, practice doing the bridge exercise and get your hips all the way up prior to pivoting over one shoulder, just as you would when you're trying to throw someone off you in the same position.

Common Preventable Injuries: shoulder dislocation, ankle sprain, neck injury, elbow injury, knee ligament sprain

Physical Demands: trunk strength, pulling strength

Goals of Program: shoulder stability, ankle proprioception, neck strength, posting strength, hip flexibility, multiplanar trunk strength, hamstring flexibility

EXERCISE	REPS/DURATION
Basic Hip Hinge, *page 91*	3 x 10 reps
Crossover Lunge, *page 100*	3 x 10 reps
Single-Leg Hip Hinge, *page 92*	3 x 10 reps
Reverse Plank Walk, *page 74*	3 x 5 reps
Power Pull, *page 120*	3 x 10 reps
Push-Up with Feet in Straps, *page 73*	3 x 20 reps
High Row, *page 61*	3 x 10 reps
Bridge (single-leg variation), *page 93*	3 x 10 reps
Prone Crunch, *page 108*	3 x 30 sec
Piriformis Stretch, *page 125*	3 x 30 sec

Part 3
EXERCISES

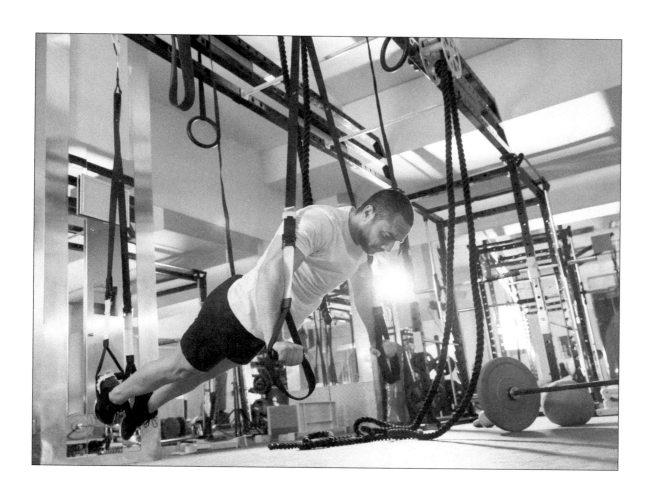

Y SQUAT

This exercise may look simple, but the difficult part is trying to keep the back and shoulders in the exact same position at the bottom of the squat as when standing.

1 Stand facing the anchor and hold an end in each hand. Raise your arms to the ceiling in a Y position and step back to remove any slack from the straps.

2 Maintaining tension in the straps, squat as low as is comfortable.

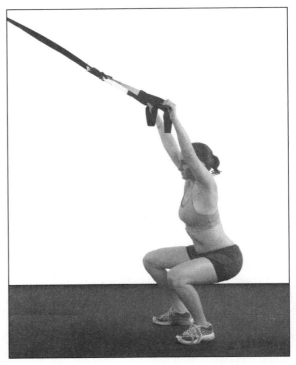

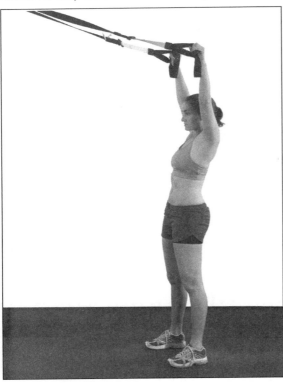

Return to starting position.

HIGH ROW

The most common compensation in any pulling exercise is to use the upper trapezius, which makes the shoulders rise up. Always try to keep your shoulders low and away from your ears. This can be very difficult, especially with the high row. When squeezing your shoulder blades, pay special attention to keeping your shoulders down.

1 Stand facing the anchor and hold an end in each hand. Step forward and lean backward, keeping your torso straight.

2 As you pull yourself upright, squeeze your shoulder blades together and keep your elbows up at shoulder level.

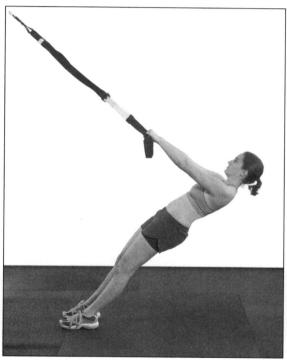

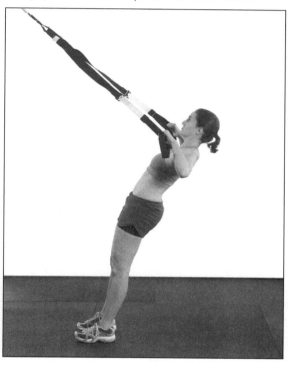

Slowly extend your arms, lowering your back toward the floor.

LOW ROW

1 Stand facing the anchor and hold an end in each hand. Step forward and lean backward, keeping your torso straight. Bend your arms 90 degrees and keep your elbows at your sides; squeeze your shoulder blades together.

2 Slowly extend your arms forward, lowering your back toward the floor.

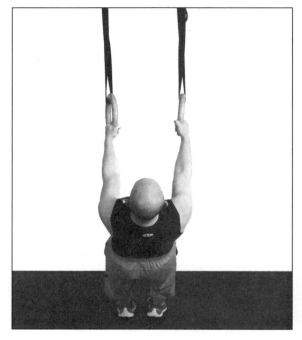

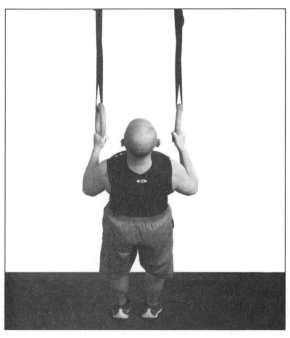

Maintaining scapular retraction, pull your elbows back to your torso to return to starting position.

SINGLE-LEG VARIATION: This can also be done with one leg off the ground.

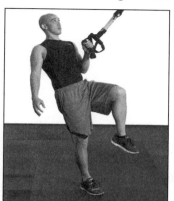

SINGLE-ARM VARIATION: This can also be done by pulling with just one arm.

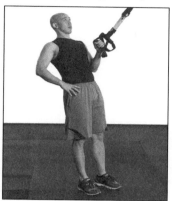

WALKOUT VARIATION: For this advanced version, attempt to take one step forward after each row. Begin to walk back up when it becomes too difficult. The deeper you go, the harder the row becomes.

X REVERSE FLY

1 Stand facing the anchor and hold an end in each hand. Take one step forward so that you're leaning back with your torso straight.

2 As you pull yourself upright, reach your left arm up and your right arm down.

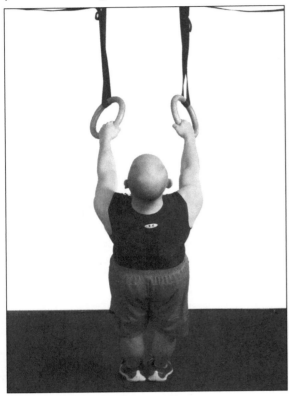

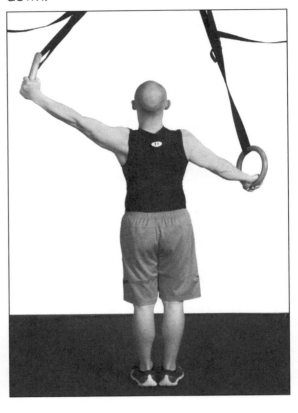

Return to starting position and then alternate sides.

CHEST PRESS

1 Stand facing away from the anchor. Grab an end in each hand and extend your arms. Step back so that you're leaning slightly forward in an upright plank position.

2 Allowing your elbows to flare to the sides, slowly lower your chest until it's in line with your elbows.

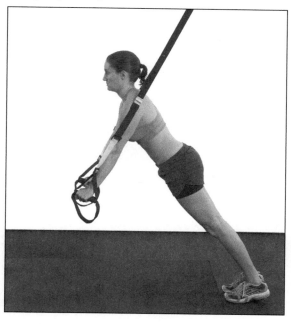

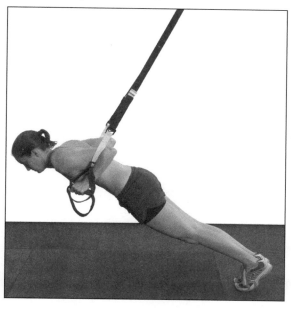

Press into the handles to return to starting position.

ELBOWS-IN VARIATION: To make it more challenging, keep your elbows by your sides as you lower.

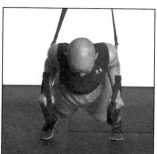

W FLY

1 Stand facing the anchor with a staggered stance and grab an end in each hand. Raise your arms up to the ceiling and then bend your elbows 90 degrees (think of a cactus).

2 Lean back and slowly allow your forearms to roll forward until they're in line with the straps.

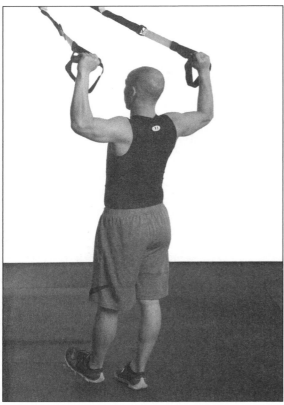

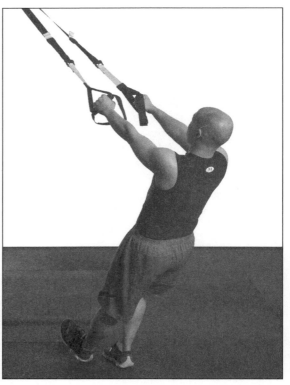

Pull your forearms back to return to starting position.

L DELTOID REVERSE FLY

1 Stand facing the anchor with a staggered stance and grab an end in each hand. Keeping your elbows by your sides, open your hands to the sides as wide as is comfortable.

2 Lean back and slowly allow your forearm to come in line with the straps.

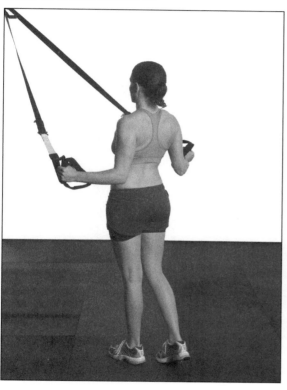

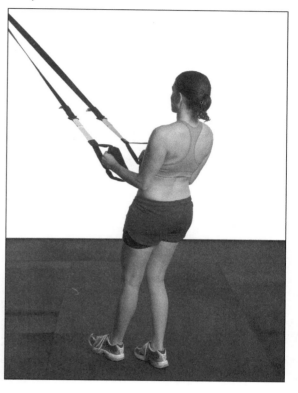

Keeping your elbows against your sides, open your arms back out to the sides to return to starting position.

T FLY (REVERSE FLY)

1 Stand facing the anchor and grab an end in each hand. Hold your arms out at shoulder height to form a "T."

2 Slowly lean back as you allow your arms to come together in front of your chest and in line with the straps.

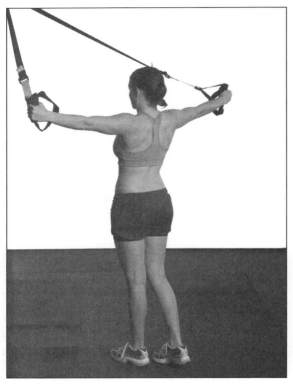

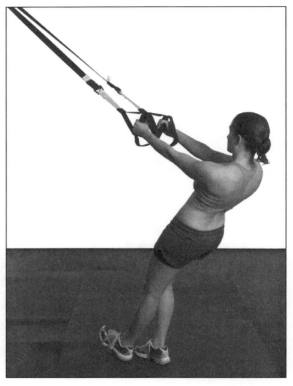

Open your arms back out to the sides to return to starting position.

Y REVERSE FLY: To increase difficulty and challenge your lower trapezius, start and end this exercise with your hands over your head in the Y position.

BICEPS CURL

1 Stand facing the anchor and grab an end in each hand with your palms up. Lean back, keeping your torso straight. Extend your arms until they're in line with the straps.

2 Keeping your elbows in place, bring your hands to your ears.

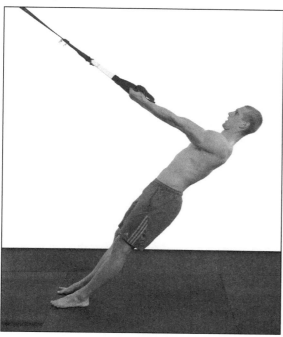

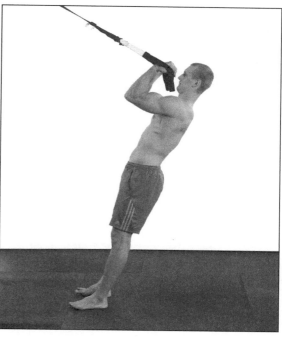

Slowly extend your arms to return to starting position.

PALMS-DOWN VARIATION: Start with your palms down instead to emphasize the brachialis.

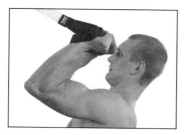

ROW AND BICEPS CURL VARIATION: Some exercises work great in combination. Try alternating biceps curls and rows.

SINGLE-ARM VARIATION: Doing this exercise with one arm makes the movement harder on your arm and increases the challenge to the core.

BICEPS-CROSSING CLUTCH

1 Stand facing the anchor and grab an end in each hand with your palms facing each other. Lean back, keeping your torso straight. Extend your arms until they're in line with the straps.

2 Bending your elbows, bring your arms in as if to hug yourself.

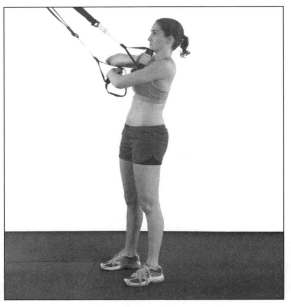

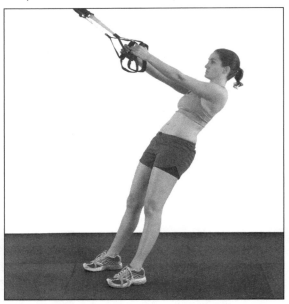

Slowly extend your arms to return to starting position. Repeat with the other arm on top.

TRICEPS PRESS ELBOW EXTENSION

Changing the length of the straps is a great way to modify the resistance. In the shortened position, you'll be more upright, which makes the exercise easier. In the fully lengthened position, the same exercise will be much more difficult.

1 Stand facing away from the anchor. Grab an end in each hand and extend your arms. Step back so that you're leaning slightly forward in an upright plank position with your arms at shoulder height.

2 Keeping your elbows in line with your shoulders, allow your elbows to bend, pointing them forward as you lower down.

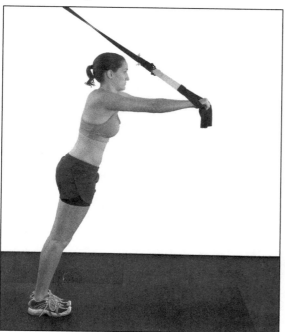

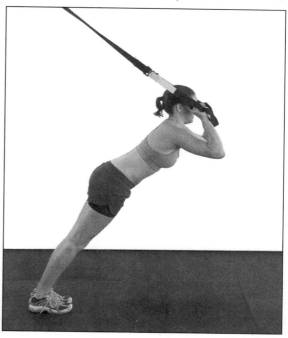

Press your hands into the handles to extend your arms and return to starting position.

OVERHEAD TRICEPS PRESS ELBOW EXTENSION

This exercise will challenge the long head of your triceps, located on the backside of your upper arm. This can help increase the overhead throwing motion.

1 Stand facing away from the anchor. Grab an end in each hand and extend your arms overhead. Take all the slack out of the straps.

2 Keeping your elbows by your ears, bend your elbows, allowing your hands to move backward.

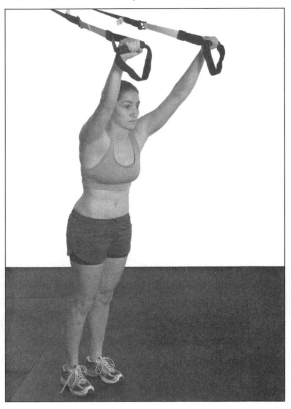

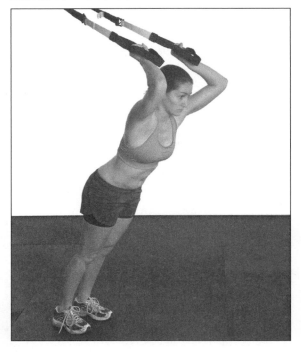

Press your hands up to the ceiling to extend your arms and return to starting position.

SINGLE-ARM VARIATION: To increase difficulty, perform this using one arm at a time.

PUSH-UP WITH FEET IN STRAPS

1 Place your feet in the straps and assume a facedown plank position. Keep your trunk tight and head in line with your spine.

2 Keeping your elbows by your sides, lower your body to the ground until your elbows are bent 90 degrees.

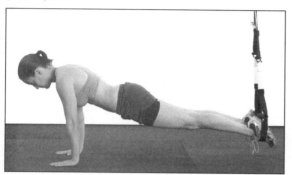

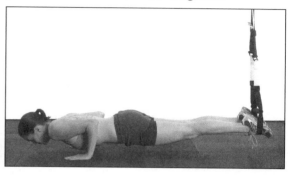

Press your hands into the floor to return to starting position.

HANDS-IN-STRAPS VARIATION: Place both hands in the straps; keep both feet on the floor.

ONE-FOOT-IN-STRAP VARIATION: Place just one foot in a strap with the other floating; keep both hands on the floor.

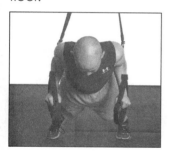

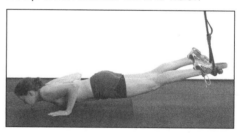

HAND-IN-STRAP VARIATION: Place just one hand in a strap and the other on the floor; keep both feet on the floor.

ATOMIC PUSH-UP VARIATION: For a great combination, try alternating push-ups and prone crunches (page 108) to challenge your arms and abs at the same time.

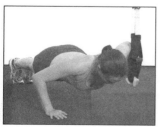

PLANK WALK

The slower you walk, the harder this is. In addition, if you're strong, you may walk yourself far back enough that your body is nearly vertical.

1 Assume plank position with your feet in the straps and your hands on the ground.

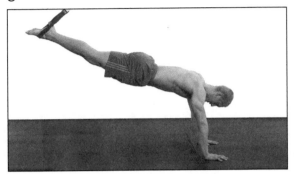

2–3 Contracting your abs to prevent any motion or sagging of the spine, slowly walk your hands backward a comfortable distance, allowing your body and legs to move in the same direction.

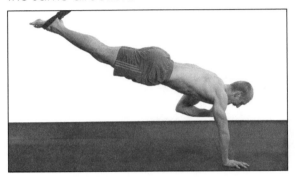

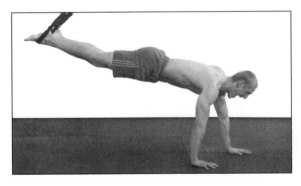

Now walk your hands forward.

PUSH-UP VARIATION: Add a push-up at the end of the walk.

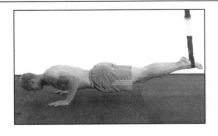

ASSISTED SQUAT

1 Stand facing the anchor and grab an end in each hand.

2 While maintaining tension on the straps, bend your knees and hips. Attempt to go as low as possible while keeping your back straight.

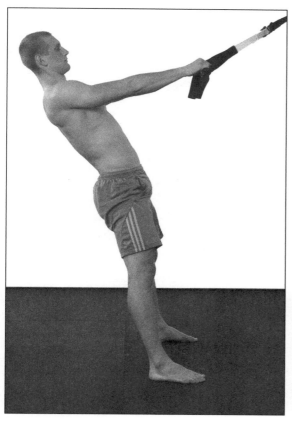

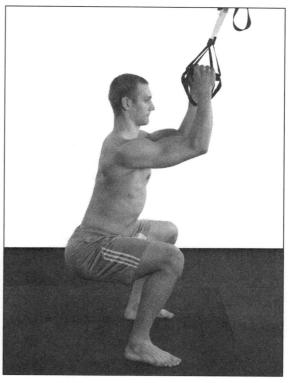

Return to standing.

FORWARD LEAN VARIATION: Another way to help with your squat is with the forward lean. Start by holding the straps underneath your armpits and facing away from the anchor. Leaning away from the suspended bodyweight trainer to maintain tension on the straps, perform the squat.

JUMP VARIATION: Try performing a jump in between reps for increased explosiveness. Make sure to land softly.

ASSISTED LUNGE

1 Stand facing the anchor and grab an end in each hand.

2 Step back with your right leg and bend your front knee as low as is comfortable.

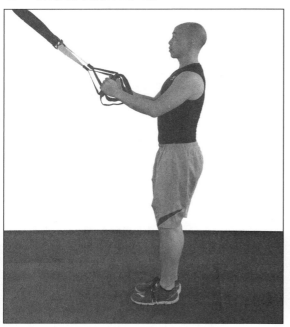

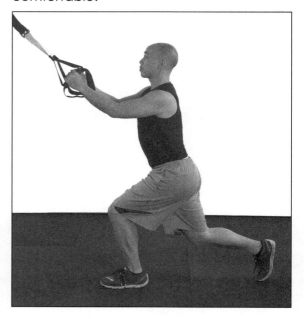

Return to starting position. Switch legs.

SUSPENDED-LEG VARIATION: For an extra challenge, keep the rear leg off the floor.

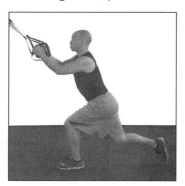

LUNGE

1 Facing away from the anchor, place one foot in both straps. Hop forward, keeping your leg behind you.

2 Allowing your back leg to reach back, lower your body until your front knee reaches 90 degrees.

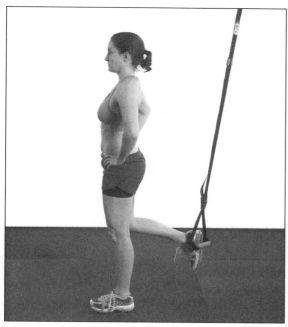

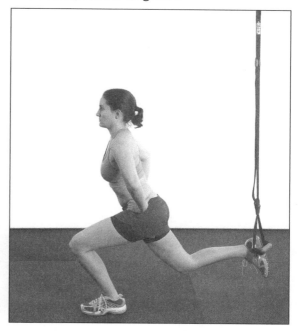

Return to starting position.

JUMP VARIATION: This can also be done with a jump. Slowly lower yourself into the lunge position. When ready, drive your rear leg forward and attempt to use your standing leg to jump off the floor. As soon as you land, allow the leg that's in the strap to travel back behind you as you control the descent.

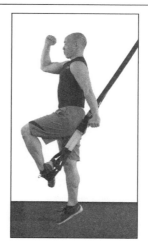

LUNGE WITH LATERAL REACH

1 Facing away from the anchor, place one foot in both straps. Hop forward, keeping your leg behind you. Reach both arms forward.

2 Allowing your back leg to reach back, lower your body until your front knee reaches 90 degrees. In addition, reach both hands to the left.

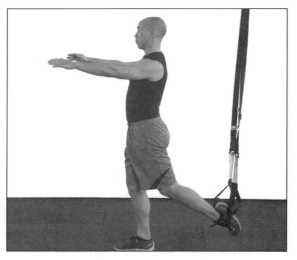

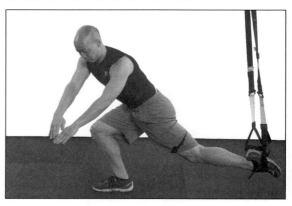

3 Return to starting position.

4 Now lunge and reach both hands to the right.

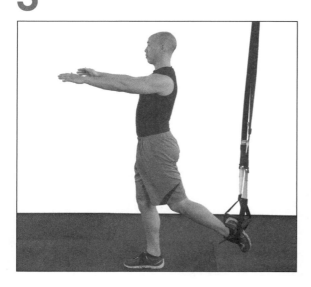

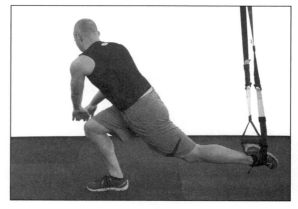

Return to starting position.

Repeat on one leg before switching legs.

LOADED VARIATION: This can also be performed with a kettlebell.

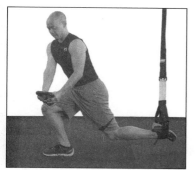

ASSISTED SIDE LUNGE

1 Stand facing the anchor and grab an end in each hand.

2 Step one foot out to the side and sit your hips back until you feel a stretch in your straight leg. Attempt to keep your knee pointed over your second toe. You can try to sink your hips as deep as you can to get a better stretch to your groin. Make sure to keep your spine straight.

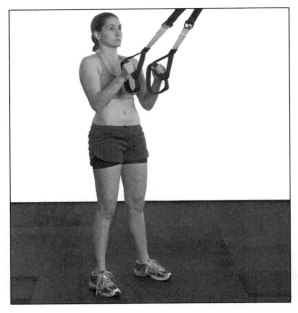

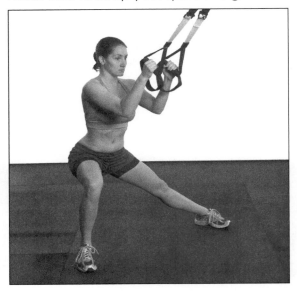

Step back to return to starting position and then switch sides.

ABDUCTED LUNGE

1 Standing sideways to the anchor, place one foot in both straps.

2 Keeping most of your weight on the standing leg, gently lower yourself as you allow the suspended leg to move sideways away from you.

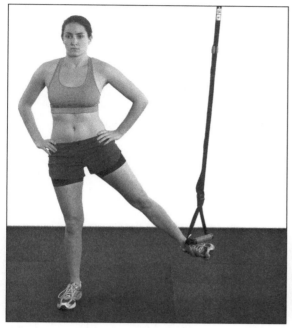

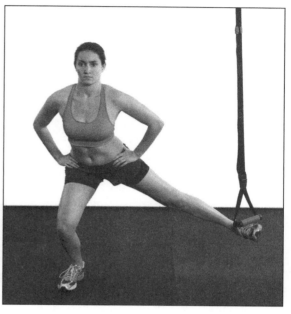

Return to starting position. Switch legs.

HEEL RAISE

1 Stand facing away from the anchor. Grab an end in each hand with the straps under your armpits and elbows pointing straight back.

2 Place your left foot in front to assist with balance. Keeping your right leg locked, press into the ball of your right foot to raise your right heel. Attempt to keep most or all of your weight on your right leg.

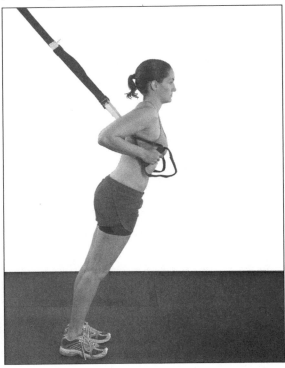

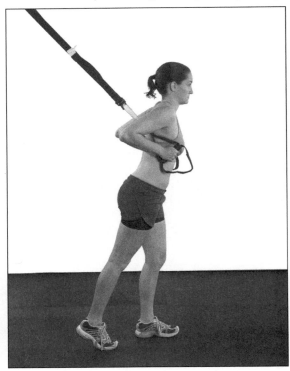

3 Lower and switch sides.

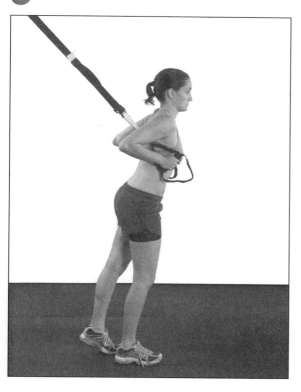

DOUBLE-HEEL RAISE: You can also raise both heels at the same time.

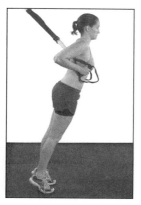

SINGLE-LEG CALF HOP: For increased explosiveness, you can perform this by attempting to jump off the floor as much as you can by using only your calves. Keep your legs straight.

FRONT SINGLE-LEG HOP

1 Stand facing away from the anchor. Grab an end in each hand with the straps under your armpits and elbows pointing straight back. Step back with your right leg until you're in a lunge position with a forward lean.

2 Drive forward with your right knee.

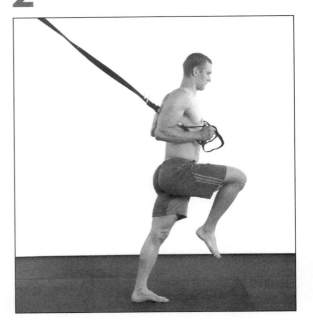

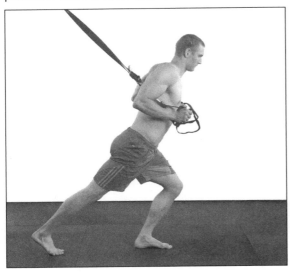

Return to starting position and switch sides.

AIR VARIATION: As you drive your back knee forward, add a little hop off your front foot. Hop back to starting position.

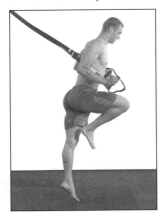

FORWARD LEAN SQUAT

1 Stand facing away from the anchor. Grab an end in each hand with the straps under your armpits and elbows pointing straight back. Lean forward and lower yourself into a squat.

2 Extend your legs.

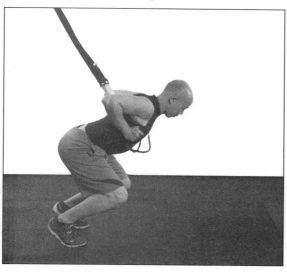

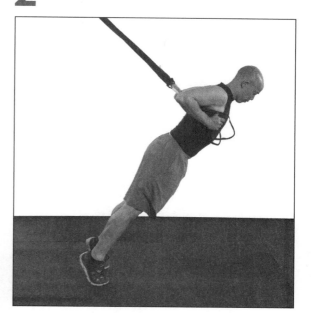

Return to starting position.

AIR VARIATION: As you extend your legs, add a hop. Hop back to starting position.

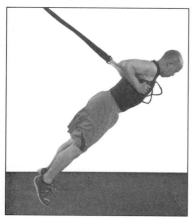

SINGLE-LEG BALANCE

THE POSITION: Stand tall facing the anchor and make sure the straps are taut. Lift one leg off the floor and attempt to keep your balance. Use as light a touch on the straps as possible; you can also try using just the tips of your fingers to help.

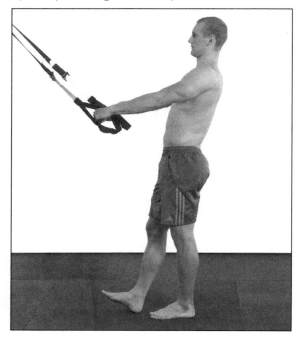

EYES CLOSED VARIATION: Close your eyes to increase the difficulty.

STANDING MARCH

This exercise can be done with different arm positions (such as with your arms over your head) to challenge the stability of your trunk.

1 Stand facing the anchor. Grab an end in each hand with your hands out to the sides. Maintain tension on the straps.

2 Keeping your balance, bring one knee up to hip height. Make sure to keep your pelvis level and trunk erect.

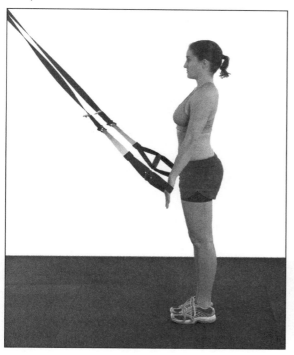

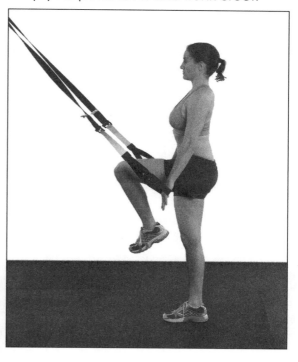

Lower your leg and switch sides.

Y VARIATION: To make this exercise more challenging, take your arms overhead.

STANDING KNEE DRIVE

1 Stand facing away from the anchor. Grab an end in each hand with the straps under your armpits and elbows pointing straight back. Lean forward.

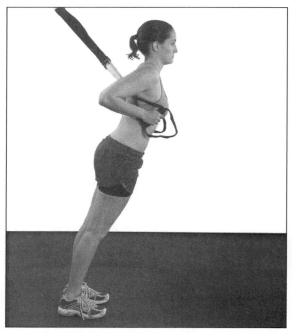

2 Drive your left knee to your chest.

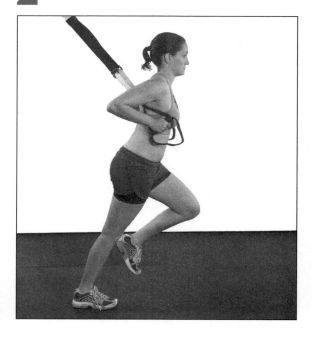

Return to starting position and drive your right knee to your chest.

Continue alternating.

CARDIO VARIATION: To increase cardiovascular work, move your knees more quickly, as if jogging or sprinting.

ASSISTED PISTOL SQUAT

1 Stand facing the anchor and grab an end in each hand. Place your right heel on the ground slightly in front of the other foot.

2 Sit back as far as is comfortable, allowing your foot to slide forward as necessary.

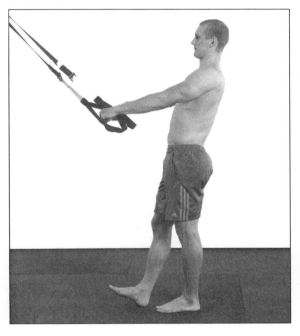

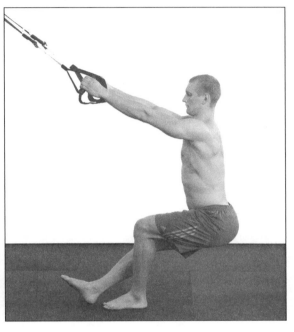

Return to starting position.

SINGLE-ARM VARIATION: For an extra challenge, hold on with just one hand.

PISTOL SQUAT

1 Stand facing the anchor and grab an end in each hand. Lift your right foot off the ground.

2 Keeping your right foot off the ground, sit back as far as is comfortable.

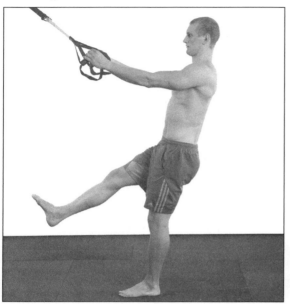

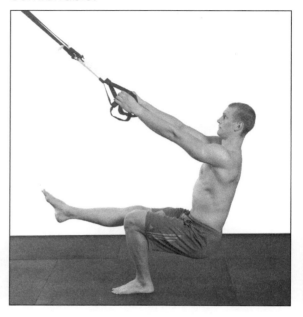

Return to starting position.

SINGLE-ARM VARIATION: For an extra challenge, hold on with just one hand.

HIP HINGE

1 Stand facing the anchor and grab an end in each hand.

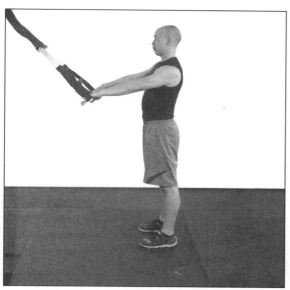

2 Keeping your back straight and maintaining tension on the straps, hinge at your hips as if performing a bow. Continue to push your pelvis as far back as possible.

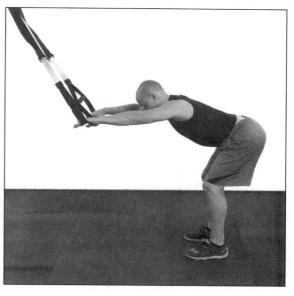

Return to starting position.

Y VARIATION: This can also be performed with your arms overhead and in line with your body from start to finish.

BASIC HIP HINGE: If you need to work on your form, do the hip hinge without equipment. Focus on bending your hips and bringing them backward (in the bottom position) and forward (when standing fully erect). Keep your weight in the same position and don't fall back onto the backs of your heels; your toes or the balls of your feet shouldn't lift off the ground.

SINGLE-LEG HIP HINGE

This exercise can be done consecutively as a strengthening and stretching exercise for the hip, or it can be held as a balance and back-strengthening exercise. Try to minimize the use of your arms when doing single-leg balance exercises like this. Instead of gripping the handles, use just the tips of your fingers, as that should be enough to help with your balance. If you need more help with balance, use something more stable than a suspended bodyweight trainer.

1 Stand facing the anchor and grab an end in each hand.

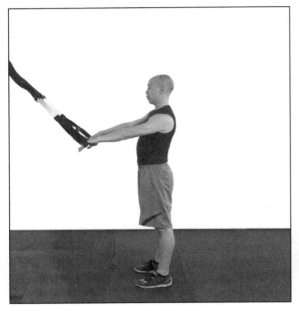

2 Keeping your back straight and maintaining tension on the straps, hinge at your hips as if performing a bow and allow one leg to raise until it's parallel to the floor. Keep your raised leg locked and in line with your upper body.

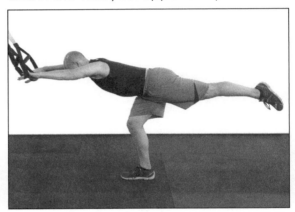

Return to starting position.

BRIDGE

1 Lie on your back and place one heel in each strap. Place your arms along your sides for support and bend your knees.

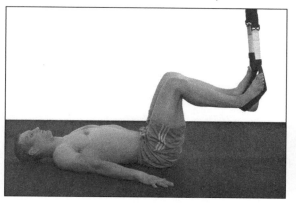

2 Press into your heels and raise your hips off the ground until they're in line with your torso.

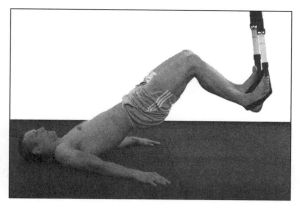

Lower to starting position.

HANDS-FREE VARIATION: For an additional challenge, do not squeeze your legs together; reach your arms up to the ceiling.

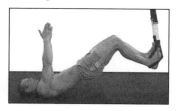

MARCHING VARIATION: This variation challenges the lower-back stabilizers. While holding the bridge position and keeping your pelvis still, "march" your legs with control by slowly straightening out one leg at a time. You can push your hands onto the floor for assistance.

SINGLE-LEG VARIATION: This can also be done with one leg at a time, either with or without your hips on the ground.

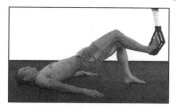

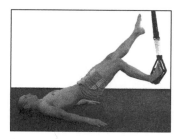

SUPINE PLANK

THE POSITION: Lie on your back and place one heel in each strap. Place your arms along your sides for support, keeping your arms and trunk straight. Do not arch your back. Keeping your upper body and hips stable, lift your hips off the ground. Hold.

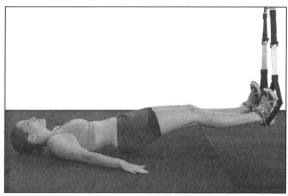

HANDS-FREE VARIATION: Reaching your arms to the ceiling makes this more challenging.

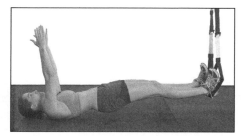

HAMSTRING CURL

1 Lie on your back and place one heel in each strap. Place your arms along your sides for support, keeping your arms and trunk straight. Do not arch your back.

2 Keeping your upper body and hips stable, bring your heels to your butt.

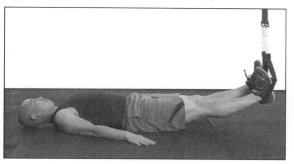

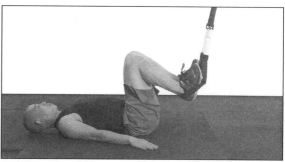

Return to starting position.

HANDS-FREE VARIATION: Reaching your arms to the ceiling makes this more challenging.

ALTERNATING VARIATION: Bring one heel to your butt at a time, alternating quickly but making sure not to rotate your pelvis.

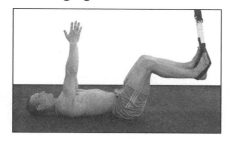

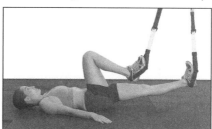

HAMSTRING CURL & BRIDGE

Perform this slowly as it may cause hamstring cramps.

1 Lie on your back and place one heel in each strap. Place your arms along your sides for support, keeping your arms and trunk straight. Do not arch your back.

2 Keeping your upper body and hips stable, bring your heels to your butt.

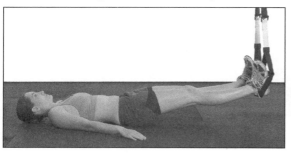

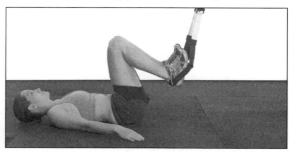

3 Raise your hips to the ceiling.

4 Lower your hips.

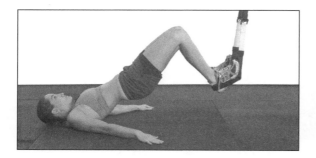

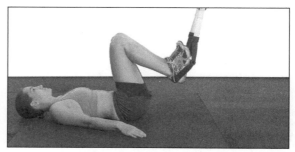

Extend your legs to starting position.

ALTERNATING VARIATION: This can also be done by alternating legs.

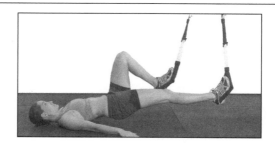

SUPINE HIP ABDUCTION

1 Lie on your back and place one heel in each strap. Place your arms out along your sides for support, keeping your arms and trunk straight. Do not arch your back.

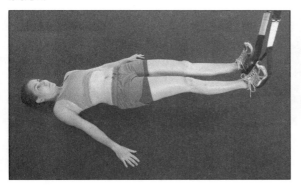

2 Keeping your upper body and hips stable, open your legs to the sides.

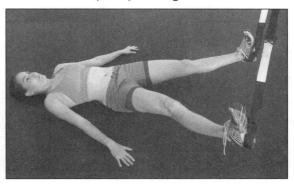

Return to starting position.

SINGLE-LEG VARIATION: This can also be done one leg at a time.

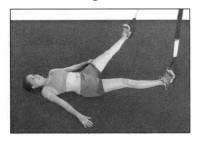

SIDE PLANK

THE POSITION: Lie on your back and place both heels in one strap. Turn to your right side, shifting your bottom leg to the back. Bracing with your right forearm on the ground, elbow directly under your shoulder, lift your hips off the ground to create a straight line from head to heels.

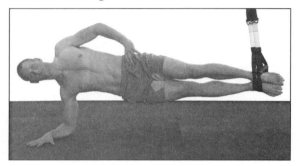

Switch sides.

MODIFICATION: For extra support, place your top foot on the ground in front of you.

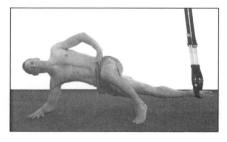

THREAD-THE-NEEDLE VARIATION: This is an excellent way to work your obliques. Hold the plank while you alternate reaching your top hand to the ceiling and then reach forward and underneath your body.

TOP-LEG-ABDUCTED VARIATION: For an extra challenge, reach your top hand up to the ceiling. You may also lift your top leg.

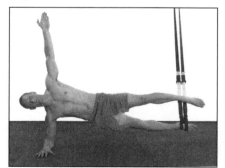

STANDING HIP DROP

1 Standing to the side of the anchor in a staggered stance (outside leg in the back), grab both ends together with your hands and hold them overhead.

2 Keeping your legs straight, drop your hips sideways to the floor. This is a very subtle movement. Try not to rotate or bend your torso.

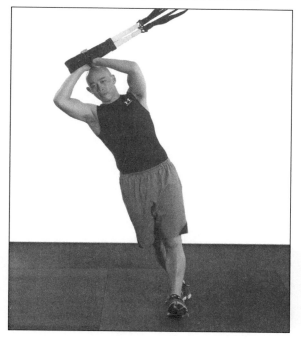

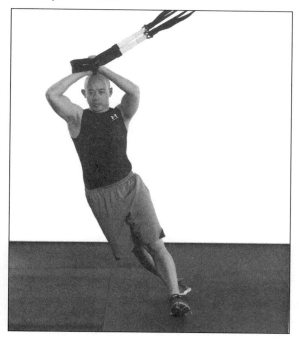

Return to starting position.

MODIFICATION: To make this easier, hold the handles at chest level.

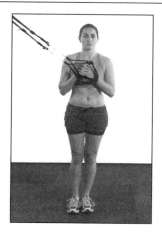

CROSSOVER LUNGE

1 Stand facing the anchor and grab an end in each hand. Step back until there's no slack in the straps.

2 Keeping your pelvis pointed forward, slide your left foot behind and across your body to the right until your right knee is bent 90 degrees.

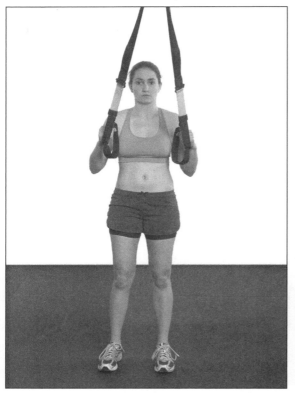

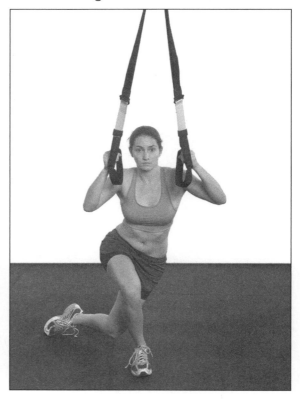

Return to starting position. Repeat, and then switch sides.

SKATER VARIATION: Perform this exercise with a slight lateral hop and switch. You'll look like a speed skater as you jump side to side with your back leg trailing behind and to the outside.

QUADRUPED HOLD

Straps should be in the low position.

THE POSITION: With your head toward the anchor, kneel and place a hand in each strap. Your arms and thighs should be vertical and your back straight. Keep your arms straight throughout the exercise. Hold, tightening your core to maintain stability. The goal here is to minimize any motion in the spine.

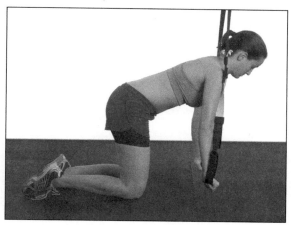

ADVANCED VARIATION: For an even bigger challenge, place one foot in each strap and assume the quadruped position with your knees off the floor.

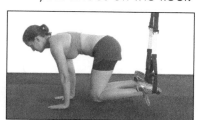

QUADRUPED WITH LEG EXTENSION

1 Assume the quadruped position (page 101).

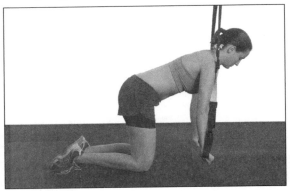

2 Minimizing any trunk or hip rotation, extend one leg behind you, keeping your foot 3–5 inches off the ground.

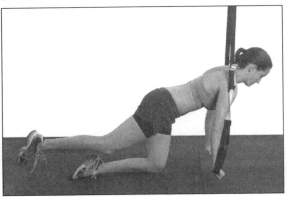

Return to starting position. Alternate sides.

MODIFICATION: Keep your foot on the ground as you extend your leg back.

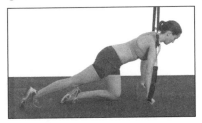

FOREARM VARIATION: Placing your forearms in the straps will make this easier on the shoulders but more challenging for the core.

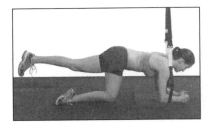

SUSPENDED QUADRUPED WITH LEG EXTENSION

1 Assume quadruped position with your left hand and your right foot in separate straps. Place your right hand on the ground beneath your shoulder and keep your left knee bent and off the ground. Tighten your core to maintain stability.

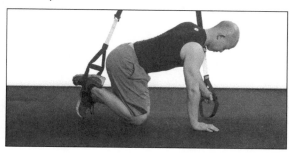

2 Minimizing any trunk or hip rotation, extend your left leg back.

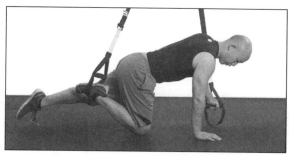

Return to starting position. Repeat and then switch sides.

ASSISTED CRUNCH

You may roll up a small towel under your lower back to help you maintain a neutral spine.

1 Lie on your back with your feet toward the anchor and a hand in each strap.

2 While maintaining a neutral spine, lift your shoulder blades off the ground. You may curl your chin to your chest or keep your head aligned with your spine.

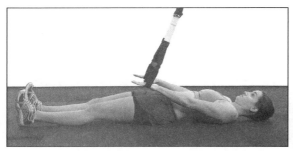

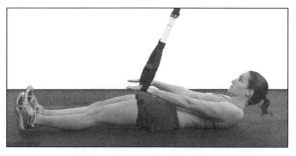

Return to starting position.

BENT-KNEE VARIATION: To increase the challenge, bend one or both knees before performing the crunch.

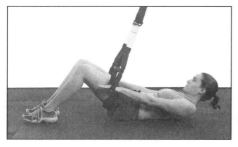

PLANK

THE POSITION: Facing away from the anchor, place one foot in each strap and place your hands on the ground so that your back is in a straight line from head to heels. Hold, maintaining a neutral spine.

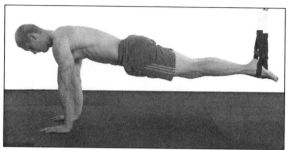

FOREARM VARIATION: If the standard plank is too challenging, place your forearms on the ground. When you feel comfortable doing this, progress to the standard version. *Note:* This is easier to do if your feet are directly under the anchor.

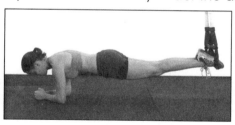

SAW VARIATION: Maintain the plank as you slowly use your arms to move your entire body forward and backward in a controlled fashion.

HANDS-IN-STRAPS VARIATION: Place your hands in the straps instead if your wrists hurt or to increase the challenge for your shoulder stabilizers.

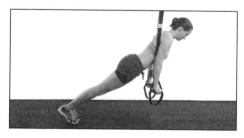

SINGLE-ARM VARIATION: Performing the plank with one arm will challenge the arm holding you up and also make your core work overtime to stabilize your body.

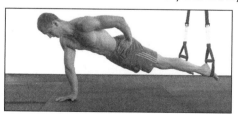

DOUBLE-LIMB SUSPENSION PLANK

If you feel stronger on one side, consider training the weaker side more often.

THE POSITION: Assume a quadruped position with one hand and the opposite leg in the straps. Keep your arm that's in the strap bent 90 degrees with your elbow at your side. Extend your leg in the strap behind you; when you're stable, lift the other leg and extend it as well. Hold.

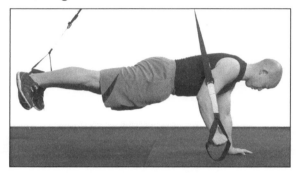

Try your best to stay still. After you feel comfortable on one side, switch to the other.

PLANK WITH HIP ABDUCTION

1 Assume plank position with your feet in the straps and your hands on the ground.

2 Contracting your abs to prevent any motion in or sagging of the spine, slowly move one leg out to the side.

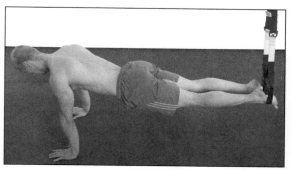

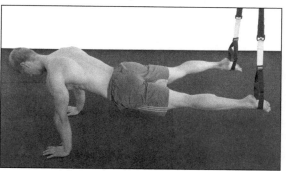

3 Return to starting position and then switch sides.

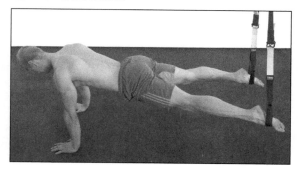

Continue alternating.

MODIFICATION: You can also move both legs at the same time.

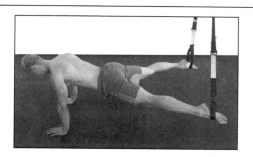

PRONE CRUNCH

1 Assume forearm plank position (page 105) with one foot in each strap.

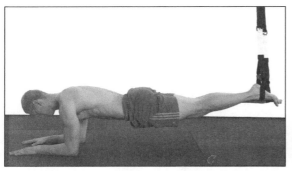

2 Maintaining neutral spine, flex your hips and bring your knees to your arms.

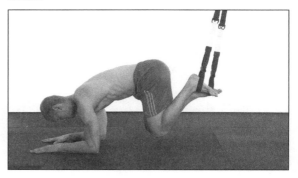

Return to starting position.

PALM VARIATION: This can also be done while on your hands.

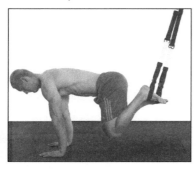

PIKE

1 Place your feet in the straps and assume the plank position.

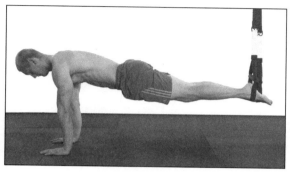

2 Keeping your back straight, reach your butt to the ceiling, letting your head come toward or even in line with your arms. Go as far as you can with control.

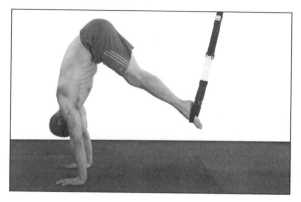

Slowly reverse the motion to return to the plank position.

SHOULDER-TAP VARIATION: For a wicked challenge, hold the pike position and then tap one shoulder with one hand without losing balance. Switch sides.

MOUNTAIN CLIMBER

A simple way to make this exercise harder is to walk farther away from the anchor. For moderate resistance, walk yourself two feet forward from the anchor point. For even more, try going out four feet.

1 Assume forearm plank position with one foot in each strap.

2 Maintaining neutral spine, flex your hips and bring your right knee underneath you.

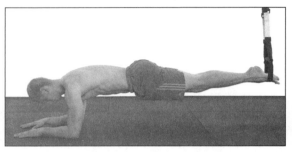

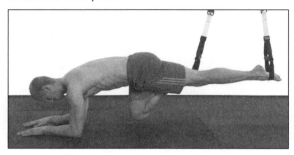

3 As the leg extends back out, bring your left knee beneath you.

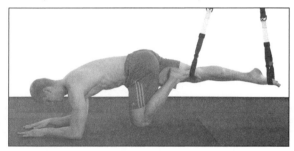

Continue alternating, making sure not to rotate or round your spine.

PALM VARIATION: This can also be done while on your hands.

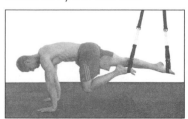

SUPINE MARCH

You could also call this the "bicycle kick" since the movement mimics riding a bike.

1 Lie on your back with your feet toward the anchor. Place a hand in each strap and bend your knees 90 degrees.

2 Pressing down lightly into the straps with your hands and pulling your shoulder blades back and down, lower one foot to the ground. Maintain neutral spine.

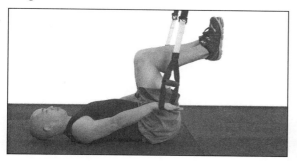

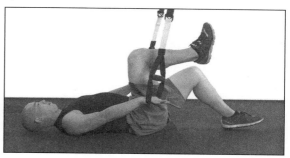

3 Return to starting position and lower the other foot the ground.

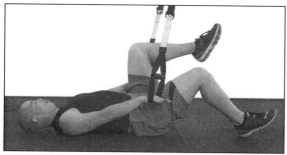

Continue alternating.

DOUBLE-LEG VARIATION: To increase difficulty, lower both legs at the same time. Make sure to maintain a neutral spine.

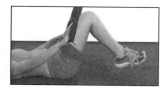

PRONE OBLIQUE CRUNCH

1 Assume a plank position with one foot in each strap.

2 Bring both knees to your left arm.

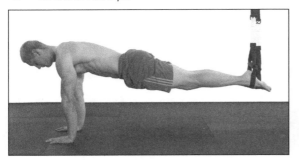

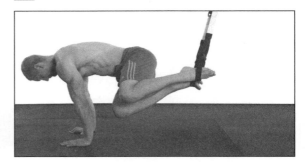

3 Return to starting position.

4 Bring both knees to your right arm.

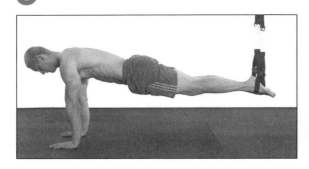

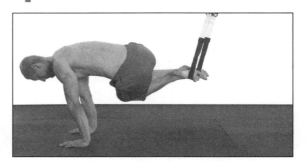

Continue alternating.

STIR-THE-POT VARIATION: Instead of returning to starting position after you bring your knees to your left arm, take your knees to your right arm and then return to starting position.

STRAIGHT-LEG VARIATION: For an additional challenge, try to keep your legs straight.

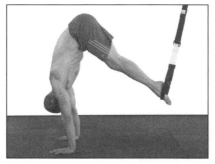

L SIT

This is an advanced movement.

1 Sit beneath the anchor with your legs extended along the floor and grab an end in each hand, bending your elbows as necessary.

2 Keeping your legs straight, hips bent 90 degrees, and torso upright, pull your entire body off the ground. Hold.

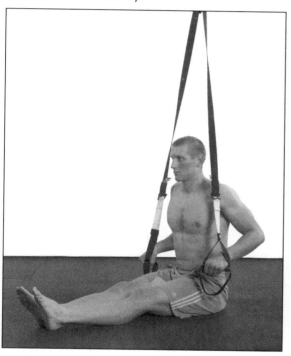

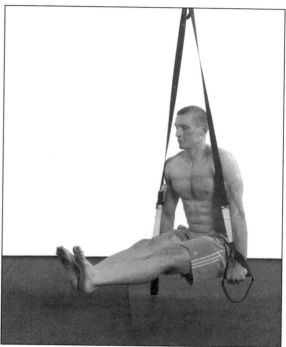

SUSPENDED KNEE CRUNCH

This exercise is done more easily with a two-strap suspension system. It can be done with a Y-strap system if the straps are fully elongated, but usually requires a higher anchor point.

1 Stand beneath the anchor and grab an end in each hand with your arms by your sides.

2 Bracing your abdominals and keeping your shoulders down and back and arms straight, bring your knees to your chest.

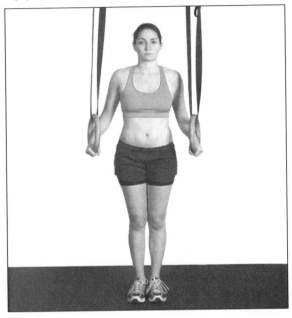

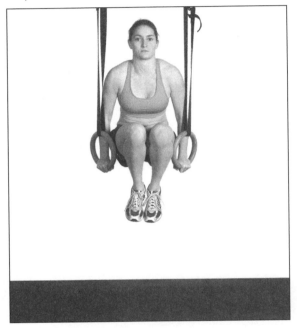

Return to starting position.

OBLIQUE VARIATION: You can also bring your knees to the side to target your obliques.

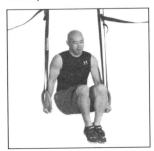

ROTATION SERIES

PUSH PULL

This is an isometric exercise so the movement should be minimal.

1 Standing to the side of the anchor in a staggered stance (outside leg in the back), grab both ends together with your hands and take them to your chest.

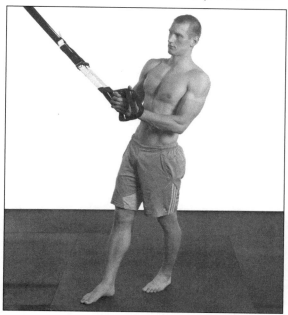

2 Keeping your legs straight, push your hands forward while preventing any movement along the spine.

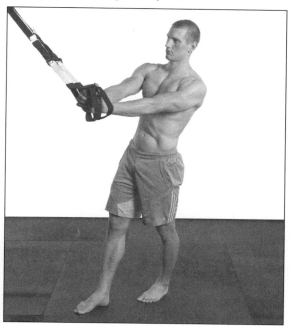

Return to starting position. Repeat, and then switch sides.

ECCENTRIC TRUNK ROTATION

1 Standing to the side of the anchor in a staggered stance (outside leg in the back), grab both ends together with your hands and take them to your chest. Keep your pelvis facing forward throughout the exercise.

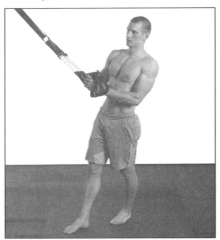

2–3 Keeping your legs straight, push your hands forward and slowly turn your chest toward the anchor as you fall away with control.

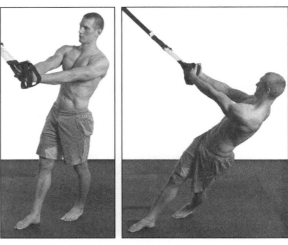

4 Pull your body back in before returning to starting position.

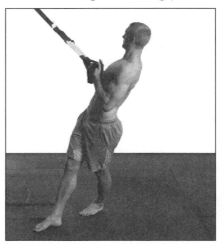

CONCENTRIC TRUNK ROTATION

1 Standing to the side of the anchor with your feet and pelvis pointing 90 degrees from the anchor, turn your chest to the anchor and lean away to take out the slack.

2 Rotate your arms and trunk until they're aligned with your pelvis.

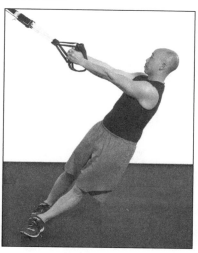

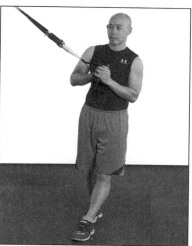

3 Pull your hands back to your chest.

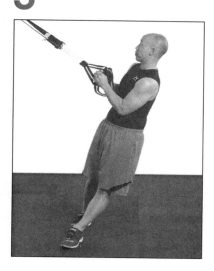

While extending your arms, rotate your trunk back to starting position.

RESISTED TRUNK ROTATION

1 Facing the anchor with a wide stance, grab both ends together with your hands and extend your arms forward. Lean away from the anchor.

2 Keeping your arms together and as straight as possible, rotate your torso and arms to the left. Your body will naturally come to an upright position.

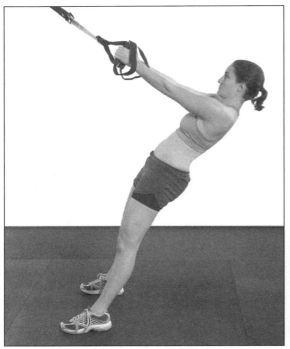

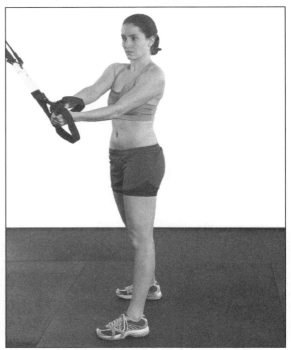

3 Return to starting position and then rotate to your right.

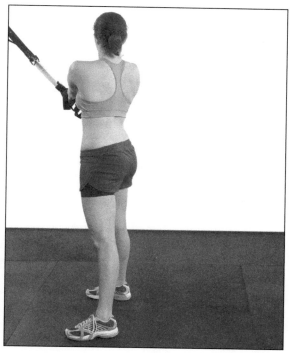

Continue alternating.

POWER PULL

1 Stand facing the anchor, grab the handles with your right hand, and place your left hand on your left hip. Take one step forward so that you're leaning back with a straight torso.

2 Keeping your weight on your heels, rotate your body to the left until your torso is in line with the straps.

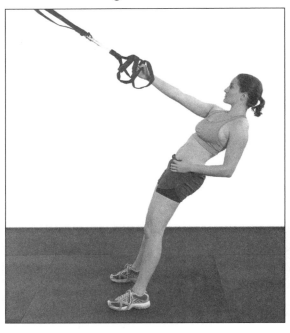

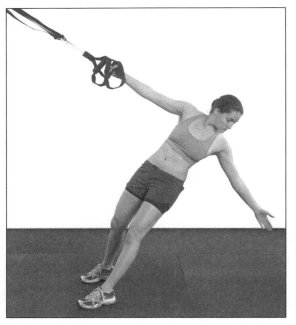

Keeping your shoulder blades retracted and your weight on your heels, return to starting position. Repeat, and then switch sides.

REACH VARIATION: As you return to starting position, pull with your right arm and reach for the anchor with your left.

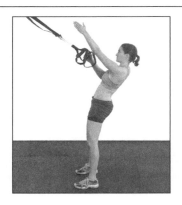

POWER PULL WITH OVERHEAD PRESS

1 Stand facing the anchor, grab the handles with your right hand, and hold a weight in your left hand by your chest at shoulder height. Take one step forward so that you're leaning back with a straight torso.

2–3 Keeping your weight on your heels, rotate your body to the left until your torso is in line with the straps. Slowly lower the weight to the ground.

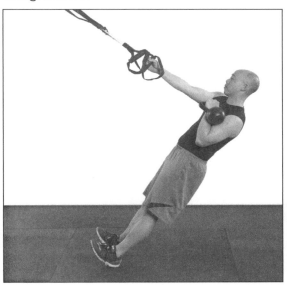

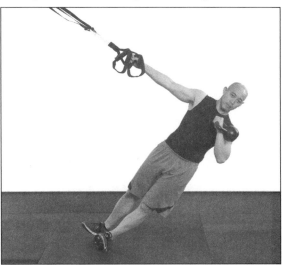

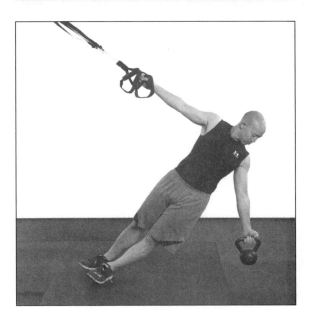

4–5 Keeping your shoulder blades retracted and your weight on your heels, curl the weight back to your chest as you return to starting position. Once you get to the top, press the weight overhead.

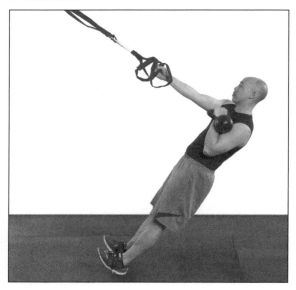

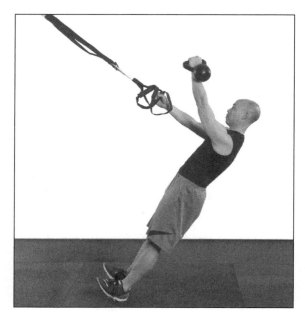

PEC STRETCH

1 Stand facing away from the anchor and grab an end in each hand.

2 Step forward with one leg and slowly press your chest forward as you squeeze your shoulder blades together.

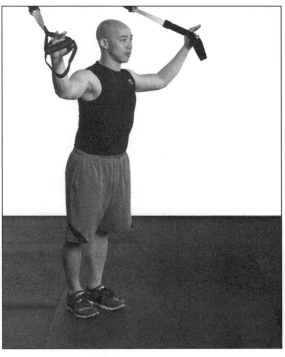

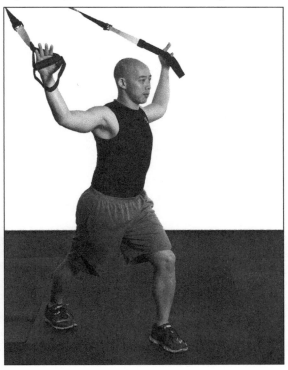

Switch sides.

REACH VARIATION: Rotate to one side and bring the back arm up.

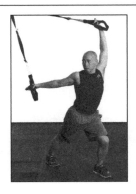

LAT STRETCH

1 Stand facing the anchor and grab an end in each hand with palms up.

2 Sit your hips back as if for a squat.

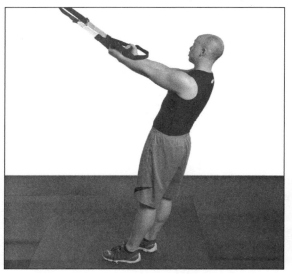

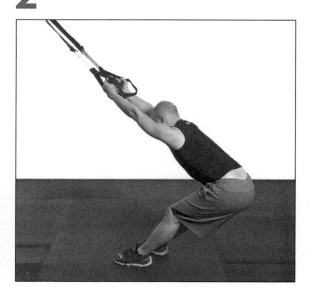

3 Keeping your left leg straight and letting your right knee bend, turn your chest to your left and look underneath your armpit. Feel the stretch in your left side.

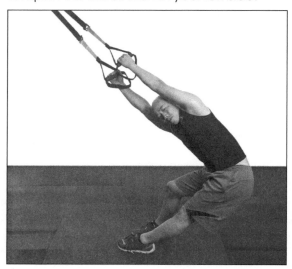

Switch sides.

PIRIFORMIS STRETCH

1 Stand facing the anchor and grab an end in each hand.

2 Place your left ankle on your right thigh and sit back as if for a squat.

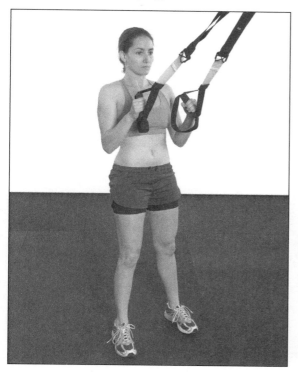

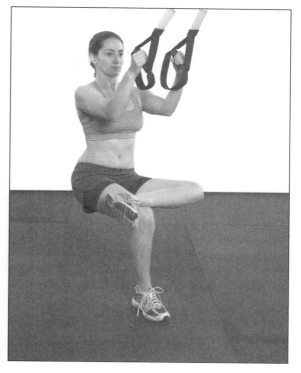

Switch sides.

LOWER-BACK STRETCH

1 Stand facing the anchor and grab an end in each hand with your palms down.

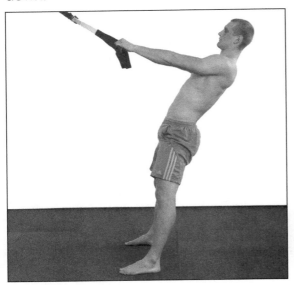

2 Sit your hips back as if for a squat.

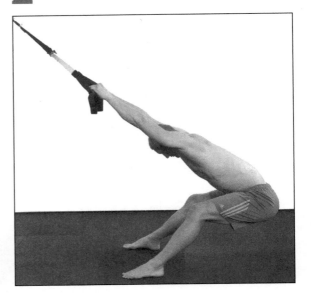

Switch sides.

TORSO TWIST

1 Stand facing the anchor with your knees slightly bent. Bend forward slightly at the hips and keep your back straight. Grab an end in each hand.

2 Turn your body and your arms all the way to your left. Allow your pelvis and spine to rotate so that your chest is turned 90 degrees or more from starting position. Hold for 1 second to feel the stretch.

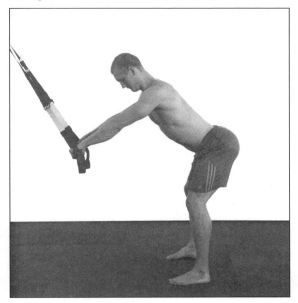

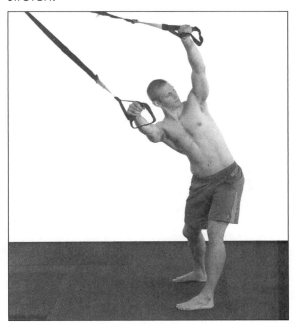

Rotate to the other side.

SINGLE-ARM TRUNK ROTATION

1 Stand facing the anchor and grab an end in each hand.

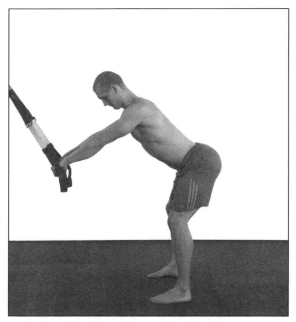

2 Keeping your waist in the same position, rotate your left arm out to the left while keeping your right arm in place. Turn your chest as far to the left as you can. You can also rotate your neck to look over your back shoulder.

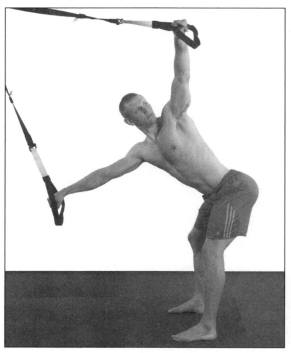

Return to starting position and switch sides.

HIP FLEXOR STRETCH

1 Kneel facing away from the anchor with one knee up. Grab an end in each hand and open your arms out to the sides.

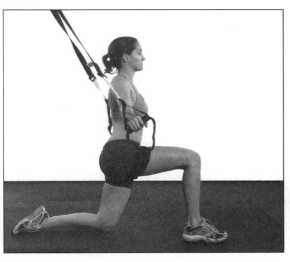

2 Tighten your abdominals and press your pelvis forward.

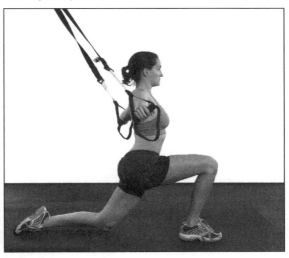

Switch sides.

TWIST VARIATION: As you press your hips forward, rotate your torso toward your front knee, open your arms, and bend to that side.

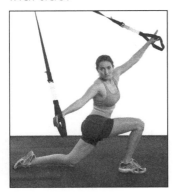

CALF STRETCH

1 Stand facing away from the anchor. Grab an end in each hand with the straps under your armpits and elbows pointing straight back.

2 Place your right foot in front to assist with balance, making sure both feet point straight ahead. Drive your back heel into the floor.

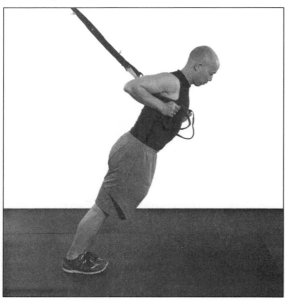

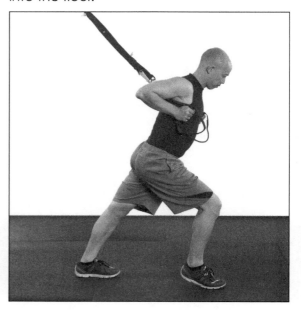

Switch sides.

SOLEUS/ANKLE VARIATION: To target the soleus more, bend your rear leg as well.

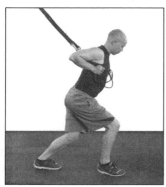

HAMSTRING STRETCH

1 Stand facing the anchor and grab an end in each hand. Step forward with one foot.

2 Keeping your spine straight, sit back, bending your rear leg until you feel a stretch in the back of your front leg.

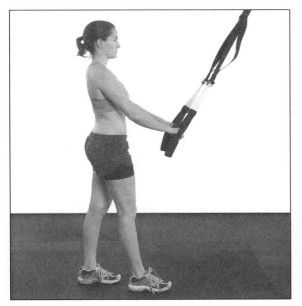 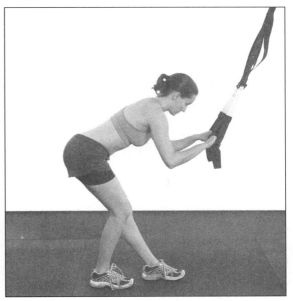

Switch sides.

NECK STRETCH

1 Stand to the side of the anchor. Place your outside arm behind your back and grab an end with that hand.

2 With the help of your free hand, bend your neck toward the anchor.

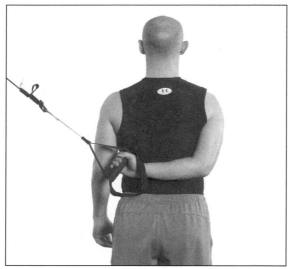

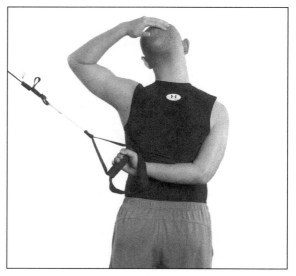

Switch sides.

BICEPS STRETCH

1 Stand facing away from the anchor and grab an end in each hand.

2 Keeping your chest open, walk forward until your arms extend behind you.

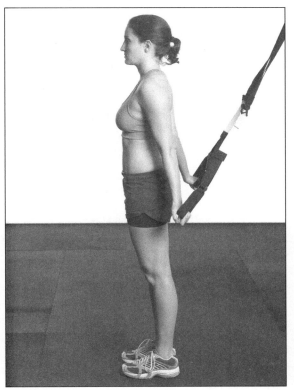

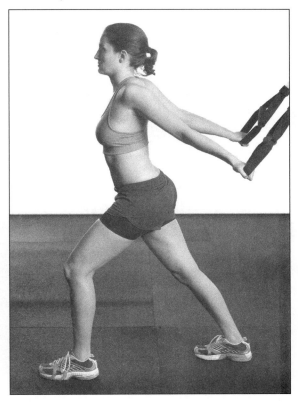

POSTERIOR SHOULDER STRETCH

1 Stand to the side of the anchor. Hold the strap with your outside hand so that your arm crosses your chest.

2 Lean away from the anchor and use your other arm to help press your elbow into your chest.

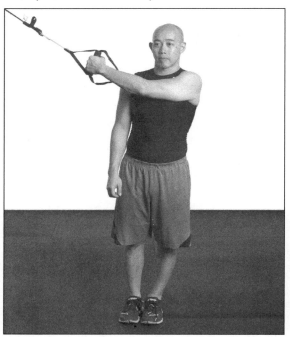

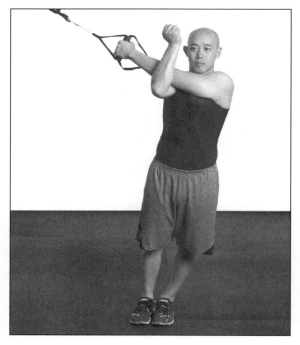

Switch sides.

PEC MINOR STRETCH

1 Stand facing away from the anchor. Hook one arm through a strap and step forward with the same-side leg.

2 Press your chest forward and turn away from the raised arm until you feel a stretch across your chest.

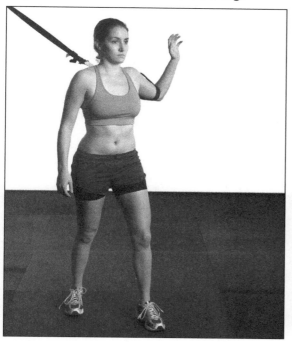 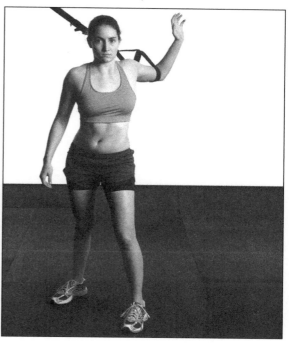

Switch sides.

INDEX

ACKNOWLEDGMENTS

First and foremost, I couldn't have done this book without my lovely wife, who continues to support me in all my endeavors while also injecting her own knowledge and opinions into our growing body of work. Thanks to my colleagues at both Sports and Orthopedic Leaders Physical Therapy and University of California, San Francisco, who continue to stay at the forefront of physical therapy and sports performance in academics and private practice. My drive to continue to grow as a health practitioner has been so much more enjoyable with all of you.

—Kenneth Leung

ABOUT THE AUTHORS

KENNETH LEUNG is a physical therapist in the San Francisco Bay Area with over 20 years of martial arts experience. Kenneth graduated from the University of California, Berkeley, with a BA in molecular cellular biology and received his doctorate of physical therapy from the University of Southern California, where he completed his orthopedic residency. Kenneth draws from his background in sports, fitness, health, and wellness to help people of all levels. He currently works with the University of California, San Francisco, and has a private practice in Oakland. You can find him on the web at www.learntomove.org.

LILY CHOU is an editor of health and fitness books, the author of *The Martial Artist's Book of Yoga* and *The Anatomy of Martial Arts*, and a martial arts practitioner. She lives and trains in the San Francisco Bay Area.